MENOPOSTAL

MENOPOSTAL

A BRIEF GUIDE TO HORMONAL SANITY

NADINE ABOU ZAHR

Copyright © 2024 Nadine Abou Zahr

The moral right of the author has been asserted.

Apart from any fair dealing for the purposes of research or private study, or criticism or review, as permitted under the Copyright, Designs and Patents Act 1988, this publication may only be reproduced, stored or transmitted, in any form or by any means, with the prior permission in writing of the publishers, or in the case of reprographic reproduction in accordance with the terms of licences issued by the Copyright Licensing Agency. Enquiries concerning reproduction outside those terms should be sent to the publishers.

Troubador Publishing Ltd
Unit E2 Airfield Business Park
Harrison Road, Market Harborough
Leicestershire LE16 7UL
Tel: 0116 279 2299
Email: books@troubador.co.uk
Web: www.troubador.co.uk

ISBN 978-1-83628-010-1

British Library Cataloguing in Publication Data.
A catalogue record for this book is available from the British Library.

Printed and bound by CPI Group (UK) Ltd, Croydon, CR0 4YY
Typeset in 11pt Minion Pro by Troubador Publishing Ltd, Leicester, UK

For Hussein and Youssef.

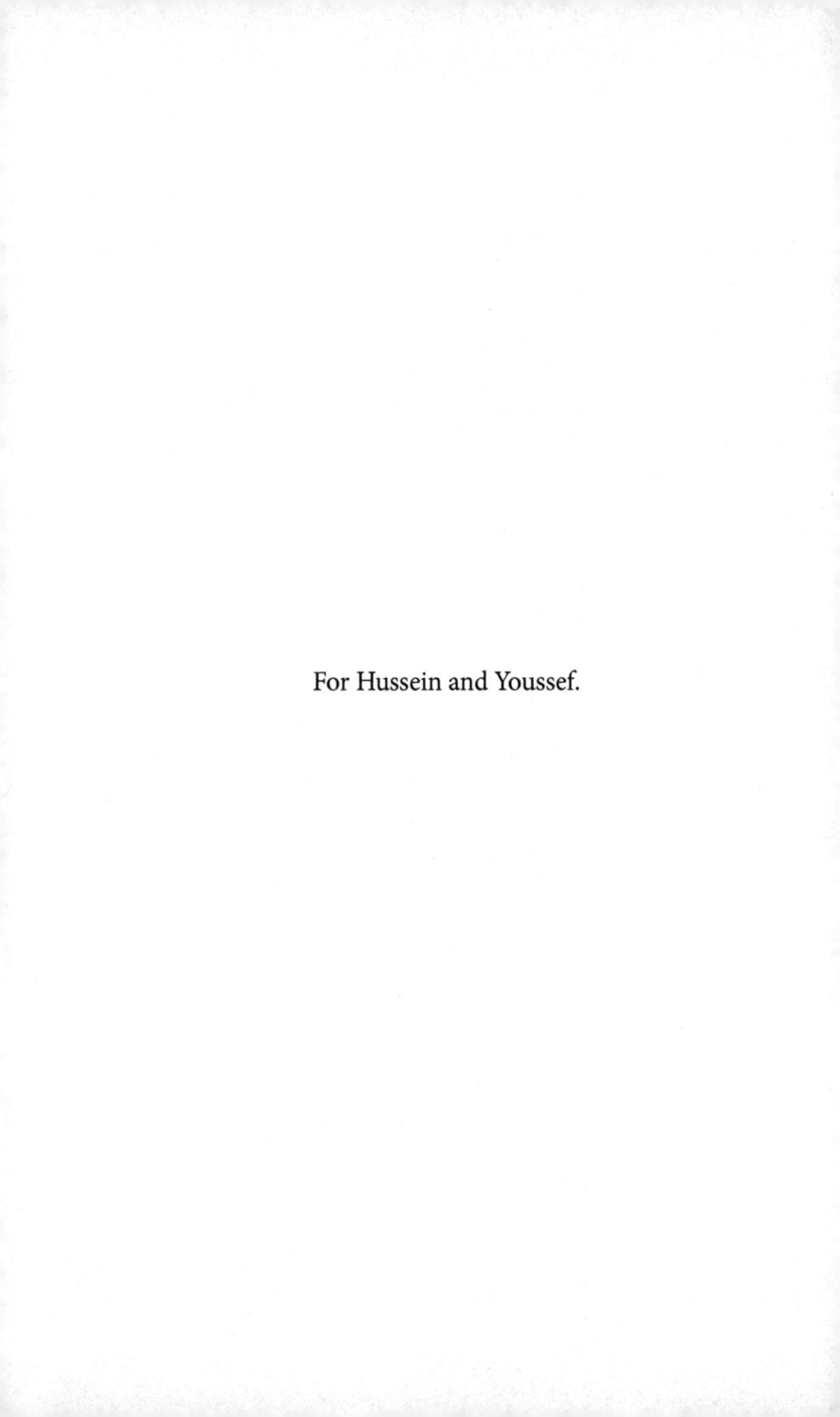

CONTENTS

NOTA BENE | 1

MENO101 | 5
HORMONAL MILESTONES | 7
MENOPAUSE DESERVES A COOL NICKNAME TOO | 10
MENOSLANG | 12
WHAT NOT TO SAY TO A MENOPAUSAL WOMAN | 14
AGE IS JUST A (BIG) NUMBER | 17
THE 'M' WORD | 19
A CONVERSATION WITH A FRIEND, CIRCA 2017 | 22
JOKE | 23

MENOBODY | 25
HELLO HOT FLASH! | 27
TRIGGER-HAPPY | 30
FUN FACT! | 32
CATCH-22 | 33
PUBLIC BATHROOM HOT FLASH MANUAL | 35
THE IMPORTANCE OF A GOOD SLEEPLESS NIGHT | 37
GOOD NIGHT, SLEEP TIGHT CHECKLIST | 40

INNER MONOLOGUE: NIGHT-TIME BATHROOM TRIP	41
GOOD NIGHT, SWEATS	43
BLOATING BUSINESS	45
WE NEED TO TALK ABOUT WEIGHT GAIN	46
BODY GLORY	48
O.S.T.E.O.P.E.R.O.S.I.S	51
AND ARTHRITIS…	53
BLADDER CONTROL TO MAJOR NONE	54
PALPITATION NATION	58
FATIGUE AND LAZINESS, POTATO POTAHTO	60
SIGHT AND SEEING AND BEING SEEN	62
MENOLOOK	**65**
BAD HAIR DAY (CADE)	67
GLORIOUS GREY	71
THE SILVER FOX THEORY	74
TEN (MENOPAUSAL) BEAUTY FACTS!	76
CHIN CHIN	78
PIMP MY WARDROBE	80
MENOLIFE	**85**
ALL THE MENOPAUSAL LADIES… PUT A LID ON IT!	87
KAMA SUTRA LIMITED	92
SEX AND THE PITY	94
TIT FOR TAT	96
MENO-MENU	99
ALCOHOL YOU IN A WEEK	100
SO I THOUGHT I COULD DANCE	103

MENOMIND — 107

MOOD SWING AND TWIST	109
NEWTON'S GRAVE THEORY	112
TOLERANCE	115
BRAIN-FOG THIS SH*T!	117
I CRY WITH MY LITTLE EYE	119
TEAR CONCENTRATION BAROMETER	121
DEPRESSION, ANXIETY AND PANIC ATTACKS	123

MENO-SILVER LINING — 125

GRASPING THE SILVER LINING	127
LA DOLCE VITA	128
NO MORE PERIODS. PERIOD.	131
A SENSE OF HUMOUR FOR A SENSE OF SELF	133
MENOPAUSE PRIORITIES 2.0	136
#JESUISKAREN	138
I PLEAD NOT GUILTY	140
VALID REASONS TO FEEL GUILTY	143
BUDDY BODY	145
THE URGENCY OF A BUCKET LIST	147
ANATOMY OF A BUCKET LIST FOR WOMEN OVER FIFTY	149
OLDER WOMEN ARE HAPPIER WOMEN	153
TO BELONG AT LAST	155
THE BEGINNING OF THE END IS STILL A BEGINNING	157

ACKNOWLEDGEMENTS	159

NOTA BENE

I had my last period at forty-one.

Until I went to see my gynaecologist for my annual check-up, I had absolutely no idea that the assortment of bizarre symptoms I'd been experiencing for months had a name. I didn't consider for a second that this absence of menstruation was down to anything other than a lot of stress and a little hormonal imbalance.

But then I got THE talk.

Dr S: 'So... N, your results came back. It seems you have what we call premature menopause.'

Me: 'OK... Is that a bad thing? Should I be worried?'

Dr S: 'Not at all – your menopause has just come a little early. It happens. Have you been feeling different lately? Maybe a little overemotional? Perhaps some mood swings?'

Me: 'It's me, Dr S. I was born overemotional.'

Dr S: 'Experiencing hot flashes, N?'

Me: 'I may have had a few unusual sweats here and there. It would just suddenly get so hot... Why? Are these hot flashes?'

Dr S: 'Yes, they are. Vaginal dryness?'
Me: 'Not dry, nope. Should I be?'
Dr S: 'Not necessarily. Good. Weight gain?'
Me: 'Oh, about that…'

Dr S is my gynaecologist.

When he walks into a room, he oozes hormonal expertise. He always looks like he just came back from a Swiss wellness retreat where he ate some baby alien's placenta, and appears very important despite also being unusually humble.

His voice is strong and confident but remarkably soothing.

Most importantly, Dr S has always respected my resourceful hypochondria, my ridiculous anxieties and my very melodramatic questions.

'Should I be worried, Dr S? It's nothing serious, right? I'm not dying, am I? You would tell me if that was the case? I can handle the truth.'

Over the past decades, he's never shown any signs of irritation even though every time I see him I hassle him with my neurotic fears and my blatant medical ignorance.

Dr S is the Hormone Whisperer.

After a longer-than-usual consultation during which he gave me a comprehensive introduction to my new hormonal status and told me what to expect now that I could no longer be expecting, I remember leaving his office feeling the same way I did the first time I got my period.

Stunned, a little apprehensive and strangely excited too.

Of all the detailed facts Dr S patiently took the time to share and explain to me, I chose to remember two points only.

No more periods.

No more babies.

I'll take that, I thought. But then, ridiculously enough, I felt…

Less of a woman. And that hurt.

I officially *menopaused* at forty-two.

At the time, for most of my female friends, menopause was a faraway land where wrinkled old ladies with white hair and aching joints clandestinely lived in shame.

The very first frustrating discovery (of many) I would make when I became a legitimate menopausal subject was that on top of the physical, mental, spiritual and hormonal chaos that had suddenly besieged my existence and my identity, I felt the obligation to remain silent. The 'M' word, as I would fast realise, was an off-limits topic that made people either terribly uncomfortable or terribly unresponsive.

At first, I really struggled to understand why. After all, even if it was happening a little early, I was just a woman going through something most women had gone through or would go through. I mean, menopause is like death. You do not skip it.

So why was I supposed to go through it on mute mode?

I chose not to.

In fact, I would reveal my expired hormonal state like a badge of honour to anyone who asked why a monsoon had suddenly materialized on my face.

I did, however, feel very isolated, because most of the women in my life and of my age were still menstruating and having babies. They really didn't mind me lamenting the loss of my hormones, my hair, my sleep and my mind, but obviously they couldn't relate to my specific misery, and when you cannot relate, you can't possibly understand.

Fast-forward ten years. Now they can.

This little book is not intended as a medical guide to menopause. There is plenty of valuable material available that will help with that and then some.

This little book, I hope, will help you navigate the tribulations of menopause with a pinch of humour, which I know for a fact remains the most powerful remedy a woman can ever possess.

MENO101

HORMONAL MILESTONES

Stage one. Before a young girl's very first period, she already understands a thing or two about the most important day of her puberty.

She knows it's scary, that it hurts; she suspects it's a little embarrassing. She has played with pads in her mother's bathroom, wondered about a tampon's exact use, gossiped about who has 'got it' and who hasn't at school, and thinks that despite its bad rap, PMS still sounds like a really cool girls' club.

And then the big day arrives. She. Gets. Her. Period. Mum gives her a little pad and a big hug, plus loving explanations and reassurance aplenty. Discreet celebration ensues, along with whispered congratulations; Dad offers a half-embarrassed, half-melancholic smile; and just like that, she's a woman now…

Stage two. Hallelujah! Our girl is pregnant! For nine months, her husband, her family, her friends, her work colleagues, the bus driver, some random woman in the cheese and dairy aisle, and her mum's Friday-night bingo group all celebrate HER (and relentlessly rub her budding abdomen on any given occasion, as if it is public property).

Congregations of ladies who all of a sudden seem to hold PhDs in gynaecology, nutrition, psychology and astrology start giving her their precious advice.

'Trust me, get an epidural.'

'Don't get an epidural, it's bad for the baby.'

'Be careful not to gain too much weight.'

'Don't forget you're eating for two.'

'Oh, it's going to be a Virgo, they're amazing!'

'My ex was a Virgo – not always easy people.'

'Girl or boy?'

'C-section or natural?'

'Breast or bottle?'

She gets more recommendations and information than her placenta can hold, but most importantly, when *the* day arrives, she is as prepared as one mum-to-be can be.

Fast-forward a few decades.

Menopause crash-lands in your life like a birthday balloon filled with liquid nitrogen.

That's stage three, by the way, and it's the last one of your hormonal existence.

You sit silently and wait.

And wait… and wait some more. And then you hear yourself internally screaming:

WHAT THE ACTUAL F***! Why on earth didn't I get the memo?!

Mum? Auntie Simone? Grandma? Doctor S? Hollywood?

Anybody?

…

And while your last hormones are bidding their farewells – *you've all been jolly good fellows, thank you very much* – the frantic questions begin to proliferate in your head:

Why is it that every morning when I get out of bed and take my first steps, I feel like the tin man from *The Wizard of Oz*?

Why on earth do I have to discover in a packed elevator between the ground floor and the seventh that menopause screws with your control centre so badly you can start crying uncontrollably and for no reason other than being in a packed elevator between the ground floor and the seventh?

What's the name of that actor again? In *Mission Impossible*… I've seen all of them. Something beginning with T…

Where is the freaking Gaviscon?

Why do I hear *boo, boo, boo* every time I walk down the pads and tampons aisle at the supermarket?

Why am I suddenly so irritated with my boss's teeth? I really wish he'd stop smiling so much.

What was I looking for again?

Why hasn't the media world ever treated this rite of passage as a cool thing? I mean, in the nineties even the heroin-chic look had its glory days. Yet menopause still can't be the new black?

Tsk, tsk…no really… Tsk, tsk.

MENOPAUSE DESERVES A COOL NICKNAME TOO

Aunt Flo, that time of the month, shark week, lady business, on the rag, my bloody valentine, the crimson tide, Carrie, the red wedding… In my lifetime, I have heard more nicknames for menstruation than I can remember. From the poetic 'Pink Lady' to the plain gory 'blood massacre', the monthly period has been a metaphor playground for almost every single woman I've known.

The list of ways to describe this notorious monthly shedding of a woman's uterine walls is as wide-ranging as it is original, and ever growing.

So naturally, I went online and typed in *menopause nicknames*.

I got an ominous, solemn hammer blow: 'The Change' – which sounded more like *The Conjuring* or *The Exorcist* than *The Sound of Music*, if you want my opinion.

I looked a little deeper and found a selection of related terms like 'mental pause' and 'menopleasing', among other menoboring expressions that in my ten years of menopause I have never ever heard anyone use.

What I realised was that women going through menopause do not use nicknames for it because they're too busy dealing with the hormonal insanity of it.

Contrary to periods, which follow a logical set pattern – PMS, period, respite, PMS, period, respite, PMS, period, respite – menopause is a flipping maze with a revelation at every corner: hot flash, irritation, crying, fatigue, fatigue, insomnia, meltdown, hot flash, hot flash, hot flash, respite, hair loss, joint pain, rage, crying fit, vaginal dryness, hot flash…

Well, the 'pause' in 'menopause' had been bothering me for some time, and I fully believed that this insufferable state deserved a nickname that would honour every single sweat droplet of it!

That's when I remembered an expression a friend would use for better or for worse:

'That's showbiz, baby!'

There's something terribly powerful about that statement: a liberating carefreeness, a subtle nonchalance, a grey-hair-don't-care mentality… and a certain control too, as though despite the inner pandemonium, you're totally on top of things.

For instance:

'You're sweating – are you OK?'
'Yup, that's showbiz, baby!'
'Oh sorry, is that a hot flash?'
'Nope! That's showbiz, baby!'
'Why are you acting crazy?'
''Cause that's showbiz, baby!'
See, you've got this!

MENOSLANG

Check-up at the doctor's. I am answering a succession of questions regarding the evolution of my menopausal symptoms while he's taking notes.

The doctor says, 'Joints?'

I naively reply, 'No, I don't smoke pot.'

He obviously didn't mean the kind of joints people smoke to relax their mind, body and soul; he meant the ones that become stiff and sore, getting in the way of your movements.

Whether we like it or not, menopause comes with a new vocabulary, and it's important to know some of it.

Words and expressions you will likely use much less now:

- Clubbing
- Jump out of bed
- I lost 5 kilos!
- Head, shoulders, knees and toes, knees and toes…
- PMS
- Turn the music up!
- Meet you there at 11pm

- Large Big Mac Combo with Coke and six nuggets with barbecue sauce
- Twister
- DJ
- Make-up sex
- PARTAYYYY
- Can I have a smaller size, please?
- Beauty sleep
- This too shall pass
- CrossFit
- Fit

Words and expressions you will likely use much more now:

- Tendonitis
- Shin splints
- Gastritis
- Organic
- MRI, CT scan
- Virgin Mary… bloody hot flushes!
- Am exhausted!
- Chopin
- Air conditioning
- Patches
- Nice walk
- Tennis elbow
- Calcium
- Scrabble
- Trapped wind
- This too shall pass
- F*** my life…

WHAT NOT TO SAY TO A MENOPAUSAL WOMAN

If the Hulk were a woman, he would undoubtedly be a menopausal one.

Exposed to anger, scientist Bruce Banner transforms into an unstoppable mean, green machine.

He consequently advises the investigative journalist chasing him not to make him angry because, he wouldn't like him when he's angry.

Exposed to anger, that is. Not hot flashes, sleepless nights, hormonal chaos, hair loss, anxiety and weight gain, just… anger.

It's fair to say that women going through menopause have an encyclopaedia of solid reasons to turn into out-of-control, brightly coloured beasts like the Hulk.

But while it's OK for Bruce Banner to switch to mean green mode because someone rubbed him the wrong way, women are expected to silently swallow a hormonal sack of rubbish and say thank you while staring at their shoes.

Well, it turns out that when rubbed the wrong way, menopause can turn some women a vibrant colour too… Carrie red.

My point is: don't make a menopausal woman angry. You wouldn't like her when she's angry…

Things you should never say to a woman going through menopause:

- Why are you sweating?
- Look at this woman, she's eighty and just ran the New York marathon.
- What is *wrong* with you?
- Have you ever considered going gluten-free?
- All women go through it…
- It's just a little weight gain.
- Shall I get you the next size up?
- It's all in your head. A good mindset is everything.
- You're not old!
- You should meditate, it really helps.
- You should join a knitting club or something, to relax.
- Just chill!
- You should try this new app for menopause…
- I saw this woman on TikTok who's also going through menopause and…
- Fifty is the new forty!
- What do you mean, you didn't cook dinner tonight?
- Why are your cheeks so red?
- You should be more positive.

- Did you sleep well last night?
- Everything is gonna be just fine.
- Have you tried Hatha yoga?
- Have you tried Kundalini yoga?
- Have you tried Ashtanga yoga?
- Have you tried Karma yoga?

And don't ever, EVER tell her to calm down! No menopausal woman in the history of calming down has ever calmed down because someone told her to calm down!

AGE IS JUST A (BIG) NUMBER

Have you ever noticed that the 'age is just a number' adage is always said by someone younger than you? Have you also observed that it's rarely meant as a fact but more as a passive aggressive remark meaning 'get a grip on yourself'?

So no, I am not *still young*.

No, fifty is not the new forty.

And no, it's not all about being young at heart either.

You can wear sneakers and listen to Lil Wayne all you want; your knee will still ache, and you will still have hot flashes if your body temperature decides that *Tha Block Is Hot*.

And if age is just a number, let's talk numbers.

- **34:** The number of symptoms of menopause, each one a debilitating force on its own.
- **51:** The average age of menopause. Just when you're done with life's assignments – kids at uni, ambition softening. Just when you're about to make peace with your life.

- **80%:** The percentage of women who will experience hot flashes.
- **5 to 14:** The number of years that menopause can last.
- **70%:** The percentage of women who will get night sweats.
- **22%:** The percentage of women who will experience insomnia.
- **18%:** The percentage of women who will have achy joints.
- **3:** The number of stages of menopause, i.e. before, during and after – same crap, different rap!
- **0:** The number of Hollywood blockbusters where the main character is a menopausal woman.
- **0:** The number of women who enjoy menopause.
- **0:** The number of non-menopausal subjects who know exactly how menopause feels.

THE 'M' WORD

I really struggle to understand why men have always been so awkward around the 'M' word.

Except for my doctor, who makes it sound like the most natural thing on earth (hold on… it IS the most natural thing on earth!), I have met very few men who could hear the 'M' word without mentally shutting their ears and internally screaming 'lalalalalalalala'.

How do I know? There's a very particular look most men share when in the presence of the 'M' word.

They blink, widen their eyes and then, realising they have let their discomfort show, give you a pinched little smile that translates to: 'I really don't want to hear your hormonal sob story, but here's a smile I hope will trick you into thinking I'm not like a regular guy, I'm a cool guy.'

But if there's one thing menopause could never take away from any woman even if it tried, it's her intuition. And her intuition is clear about the fact that men and menopause are like baking soda and vinegar: they don't mix. They just don't.

It's as if we're talking about an everlasting bloodless menstruation – the 'M' word makes them uncomfortable and slightly nervous because they genuinely have no idea what to say or think about it.

Most people don't care about menopause not because they are apathetic jerks, but because unless you're a hormonal empath, it's really difficult to relate to something you don't comprehend. And menopause, let's admit it, is hard to comprehend even for women going through it!

This lack of understanding applies to women too. And what non-menopausal women won't display in discomfort, they will make up for in indifference.

You need to bathe in the menopausal swamp to appreciate and weigh up the implications, losses and madness that this complex chapter involves.

Menopause is a little like divorce. Unless you've been through it, it is almost impossible to understand the ferocity, the agony and the grief that comes with it, because it is such a personal and intimate journey.

Mea culpa, but until my doctor sentenced me to life without hormones, I wasn't even remotely curious about that condition where you couldn't have babies or periods anymore.

I didn't care.

I didn't even pretend to care.

And most women don't either, until menopause comes ~~knocking on~~ kicking down their door.

I do, however, believe there is something else that triggers the obvious discomfort some men reveal when you say the 'M' word.

Our vulnerability in the face of time.

Because menopause is not just a word or a sequence of maddening symptoms – let's face it, it's also an end.

It's the end of a woman's hormonal life, her vigour, her sensuality, her bloom.

It's saying goodbye to fundamental fragments of her identity.

It's accepting and gradually welcoming a new chapter in which many of the attributes that defined her as a woman up until now must be left behind.

Most importantly, it's taking a step towards the beginning of the end.

And why would men feel unconformable about that?

Well, maybe because by proxy, they fear they are doing the same.

A CONVERSATION WITH A FRIEND, CIRCA 2017

'So how does it really feel? Menopause, I mean?'
'Hmm, OK… when did you last get your period?'
'Today is my first day, actually.'
'How are you feeling?'
'I feel great! Deflated, back to normal, so relieved.'
'How about yesterday? How did you feel yesterday?'
'Oh my God, horrible, I was dying – like a time bomb ready to explode. Seriously, I was going nuts.'
'Now imagine being stuck in that state you were in yesterday for the next two to seven years.'
'WTF?'
'Yes, that's exactly how it feels…'

JOKE

Three menopausal women walk into a bar.

MENOBODY

HELLO HOT FLASH!

If, before menopause became a thing I had to care about, you had asked me what a hot flash was, I probably would have said that it's when a woman has a sudden flashback to a steamy night she once shared with a tall, dark stranger.

Ask me again today, and I'll tell you that the only steamy thing about a hot flash is your menopausal face.

A woman's first hot flash is one she can hardly forget. It's like an unexpected crush… except the crushing happens to your dignity.

Case in point.

My first hot flash is one I will deeply and forever treasure. (Deep, deep in my subconscious mind… no, deeper.)

I was a journalist in Paris, sitting in a chic conference room near the Place Vendôme, waiting to interview the owner of a famous French brand.

The questions I had prepared were smart; I was elegantly dressed for the occasion; and I was in a particularly confident, cheerful mood that day.

My *très* handsome interviewee walked in with his assistant. He greeted me warmly, took a seat across the table from me, and after brief Parisian trivialities, the interview began.

Everything was going to plan. He seemed to appreciate my questions, I was eloquent – which I'm not always – and we even shared a few *haha*s.

I was already internally gloating about a journalistic job well done.

Of course, this was exactly when my first menopausal drop of sweat decided it was time to roll. I wiped it away discreetly, hoping my gentle dab would go unnoticed, when all of a sudden it felt as if my whole head had been shoved into a custom-made sauna. A monsoon of sweat droplets appeared on my face, which I obviously couldn't ignore anymore. The real problem, however, was that neither could the two alarmed spectators in the room.

The gentleman uncomfortably handed me a tissue to wipe my Aquaman face; the young assistant looked confused and asked me if I was OK. Meanwhile, I was resolutely staring at the vase on the white marble table and wondering: 'If I take out the white roses and shove my disgraceful head into the water instead, will it fit through the opening? Will it cool off?'

Instead of burying my head in the vase, ostrich-style, I opted for drama; I struck a theatrical pose (think Debra Winger in *Terms of Endearment*) and answered: 'No, I'm not feeling too well, actually. I don't know what's wrong with me… I feel dizzy.'

Apart from the facial sweat party, I was perfectly fine, but I had to justify this sudden perspiration and so

I decided to lie, buying myself a few minutes to 'compose myself' and leave.

Needless to say that, as I left the office and slowly drifted towards the lift, right before my two witnesses' puzzled eyes, the walk of shame took on a whole new meaning for me.

As soon as I got into the lift, the glorious secretion that had just ruined my interview, my ego and my day completely stopped. Timing really is everything.

I was a little perplexed and *a lot* embarrassed, but decided that this regrettable humiliation was probably a bizarre, isolated incident.

Menopause: 'Hold my drink!'

TRIGGER-HAPPY

List of hot flash triggers:

- Red wine
- Coffee, cappuccinos and lattes
- Spicy food (think a really good Thai curry)
- Relaxing hot baths
- Hairdressers
- Your favourite dessert
- Emotions
- Good sex

List of hot flash non-triggers:

- Steamed broccoli
- Porridge
- Herbs
- Salmon (not the kind you find in supermarkets; the expensive one you can't afford)
- Water
- Staring at a blank wall

It's as if menopause made a list of all the treats a woman relishes, the things that keep her going, that help her unwind or recharge… and said, 'Hey, let's turn these gratifying small pleasures into hot flash triggers – it'll be fun.'

And as if that wasn't enough, on a last-minute sadistic, misogynistic whim decided: 'And how about I throw EMOTIONS into the mix! Now, won't *that* be entertaining?'

FUN FACT!

Did you know that some women can experience a recurrence of hot flashes more than ten years after menopause, even into their eighties and beyond?

While some women, born under a lucky star, barely experience any hot flashes at all, others can actually take them to the grave.

You should also know that the duration of a hot flash is unpredictable. It could be two minutes or four minutes; it could be ten minutes.

Once the dreadful upper-body sweating fiesta begins, nobody knows how long it will last, and whether it will come back in half an hour, next week, or never again.

Nobody. Not you, not your doctor, not Oprah, not even Nostradamus: nobody.

So, if you're looking for an estimate of when the mad sweating will stop completely, death might be the best guess.

You're welcome.

CATCH-22

If you're at the gym, lost in the middle of the desert or in a sauna, you are expected to sweat. This is called Regular Sweat – it's healthy; it's normal; it's your body regulating and cooling itself in response to physical effort or a sizzling environment.

Outside these circumstances, however, sweating is a whole different story.

Introducing Stress Sweat: the kind where your body reacts to an emotion like anxiety, shame, fear or unease… AKA Humiliation Sweat.

This type of perspiration is always looked down on and frowned upon, and non-sweating people will often associate it with someone who can't control their emotions or has something to hide; in other words, someone who's either weak or can't be trusted.

It's unfair and demeaning, but so is life sometimes.

And then you have menopausal sweat. Your newfound sweat. The kind of sweat that's associated with everything and nothing.

The kind of sweat that usually likes to focus on your face, because let's admit it, where would the fun be in having your ankles drip?

Now... Imagine you're in a restaurant surrounded by friends and acquaintances, when suddenly it's hot flash o'clock.

What do you do? What do you say?

Because most people are nosy parkers and even if they remain silent, their wide-open eyes and mouth demand an explanation, and a rational one too. They need to know why your skin is unexpectedly singing 'Raindrops keep fallin' on my face', and they need to know NOW!

So... here comes the sweet sweat dilemma. Do you tell them you are dripping everywhere because you're a nervous wreck and can't control your emotions, or do you choose to share your hormonal expiry date, along with all the miserable details it implies?

Well, it turns out you don't have to do either.

Meet Public Bathroom, your new best friend and hot flash time-out space.

PUBLIC BATHROOM HOT FLASH MANUAL

As soon as you feel the tropical heat mounting, excuse yourself and walk straight to the bathroom. Try to look casual; don't display any sign of panic, frustration, embarrassment or *Oh shit, you again...* Act normal, I repeat act normal, like you're going to the bathroom to powder something or throw up your fried calamari.

You're in the bathroom now.

1. First, pull a few paper towels from the dispenser and thoroughly wipe your face (waterproof mascara would be a good investment now), your neck, and any part of your body in need of towelling.
2. Once this is done, turn on the cold water (obviously), run your hands under it and pat your face delicately. Don't just splash water on your face because you might wet your top by accident or ruin your makeup. We don't want that.

3. Then, wipe your face again with another paper towel until it's dry.
4. Finally, let your hands cool down under the running water for a few minutes, or until your body figures out what flipping temperature it should be at. (Don't worry about the paper towel and water consumption; we'll save the planet later…)
5. Once your body remembers it's winter and snowing outside, nonchalantly walk back to your table and immediately divert attention from your return with a gossipy comment:

'You're not going to believe it. I just saw Elon Musk on my way to the bathroom. I didn't know he was so tall.'

Between Tesla, SpaceX, Twitter, and everything else this man's portfolio holds, nobody will notice that you just spent eight minutes nursing your hot flash in the bathroom!

THE IMPORTANCE OF A GOOD SLEEPLESS NIGHT

A few years ago, in a bid to self-help and upgrade my then borderline-acceptable menopausal *zzz*, I bought a book written by a scientist and professor of neuroscience and psychology, specialising in sleep.

The title of the book, along with the great reviews it had scored, sounded important enough for me to trust that I was going to acquire some vital nocturnal information – which would hopefully help me sleep like a baby again.

Truly wishful thinking.

In this book, I discovered that you can eat healthily, do sports, not smoke, not drink, not stress, but if you do not sleep for seven to eight hours a night, *you're toast*. That's it.

Period.

No buts.

What started off as a book full of promises and hope, one that was going to fix my nightly glitches and help me wake up fully rested and refreshed, gave me a real complex, leading me to develop full-on insomnia and anxiety about the ravaging effect of the lack of sleep I had developed after reading it.

I mean *come on*: if you want someone to sleep, you don't tell them 'Sleep or else!' Their brain will instinctively run to the *or else* option. Fact.

If someone tells you 'Don't look up!', are you going to look left or right or down or sideways?

No.

You're going to look up, and you're going to look up pronto!

Where is the neuroscientist's reverse psychology here?

And so began a month-long journey of desperately trying to unlearn the material I had absorbed about snoozing, dozing, catnaps and siestas.

I watched TV until I fell asleep most nights, with my phone comfortably resting on my chest; ate a comforting snack right before doing so; and adopted an *if I'm going down, I'm going down in flames* attitude.

Eventually, that tactic – combined with the memory fog I had developed – helped me resume my tolerably inconsistent sleep, thank you very much.

I did, however, retain a few fascinating facts.

I finally understood why we shouldn't eat before going to bed. (Yes, it took me that long to ask myself why.) It's because, if we do, our system will be busy digesting the food we have eaten, instead of regenerating our body and mind, and fixing stuff like grouchy moods or recurring joint pain.

I understood why the temperature of the room you sleep in is important, plus why and how meditation and breathing help, among other interesting facts.

But in the end, I came to the conclusion that sleep after menopause is not something I will ever be able to control.

No matter how angry or exhausted I am.

Sometimes, I will apply all the rules Mr Neuroscientist recommended and still have insomnia beat me to a pulp.

Other times, I will eat, drink and do the opposite of every single thing prescribed on the good-night's-sleep list, and miraculously enter the land of nod from the get-go. Even better, I will wake up feeling like some miraculous intervention re-energised, recharged and restored me during the night.

In conclusion, my very personal opinion on the matter is inspired by a man who may not be a scientist and professor of neuroscience and psychology specialising in sleep, but seems to have understood a thing or two about life and everything nice. His name was Forrest Gump and he compared life to a box of chocolates. Menopausal sleep, I guarantee you, follows the same principle.

GOOD NIGHT, SLEEP TIGHT CHECKLIST

- Keep your bedroom at a comfortable temperature. √ (-5°? Done!)
- Brush your teeth. √ (Of course!)
- Wear comfortable sleepwear. √ (Easy.)
- Listen to soothing sounds. √ (I've got this!)
- Be positive. √ (Let's do this!)
- Meditate. √ (OK… I'll try!)
- Close the shutters. ∜ (Don't have any.)
- Don't eat for four hours before you go to bed. ∜ (What do you mean, four hours?)
- Stay away from caffeine. ∜ (Does chocolate count as caffeine?)
- Don't use your phone in bed. ∜ (What about iPads?)
- Avoid napping in the afternoon. ∜ (Like I can control it.)
- Don't drink alcohol before going to bed. ∜ (Why?)
- Be consistent. ∜ (Define consistent.)
- Try to relax. ∜ (YOU try to relax!)

INNER MONOLOGUE: NIGHT-TIME BATHROOM TRIP

Perfect… just perfect. Best position ever. My whole body is so happy right now. Oh, I should memorise this position so I can recreate it. So comfy… duvet, pillows and mood all aligned for a perfect night's sleep. Woohoo!

…

Ughhh… no… no… please, no.

I just went like ten minutes ago. Emptied my entire bladder.

Not now – this is just so snug.

I don't care, I'm not moving.

I won't. Screw it. I'm way too comfortable.

Control. It's all in the mind. Surely it can wait until the morning.

I mean, what if I can't find this exact position when I come back? It's so warm and comfortable.

Nope, no, negative. Not moving.

I'm way too relaxed.

...

Or maybe if I went, I would feel even more relaxed. Like, totally relaxed.

But what if I don't? I mean, I'm almost asleep.

OK, I need to pee. I think I really need to pee. Maybe it will be better if I just go to the bathroom. Get it over with.

Like, I could be totally hassle-free right now. I wouldn't have to think about going to the bathroom anymore.

I'm almost asleep, though. If I get up now and turn on the light… if I move, I might fully wake up again. I might not be able to find that perfect position again, let alone fall asleep.

I was virtually there. Dozing off, almost REMing and all.

It's so cold.

...

F***ING BLADDER BULLSH*T!
FINE! I'M GOING, I'M UP NOW.
BLADDER EMPTY… AND I'M WIDE AWAKE.
HAPPY?

GOOD NIGHT, SWEATS

Night sweats are hot flashes, but the kind that happen at night. You know, in case they didn't wear you out enough during the day.

As you may know, an individual's sleep is divided into four phases: N1, N2, N3 and REM.

- N1: Non-REM sleep. Occurs when you first fall asleep.
- N2: Non-REM sleep. This stage involves the light sleep just before deep sleep.
- N3: Non-REM sleep. In stages 3 and 4, deep sleep begins and so does the restoration of body and mind.
- REM: Rapid eye movement sleep, AKA dreams.

Now, guess which stage of your night these menopause sweats choose to disrupt?

...

No really, take a wild guess.

THE MOST RESTORATIVE ONE. The stage that is supposed to fix the things menopause has destroyed, if only menopause would let it.

I swear you couldn't make up this stuff up if you tried.

Also, night sweats are known to create nocturnal havoc between heterosexual couples, because for some unexplainable reason, men refuse to sleep in rooms with a temperature of minus ten degrees. (Look up: IKEA GRÖNLID 3-seat sofa-bed with chaise longue.)

BLOATING BUSINESS

Every human being has experienced a bloating episode or two at some point in their lives, where the stomach feels tight and full and stretched, and you are desperately trying to find an emergency exit for that excess air trapped in your stomach.

Bloating is uncomfortable, annoying and frankly quite awkward.

During menopause, bloating occurs – because why wouldn't it?

As changing oestrogen and progesterone levels slow down the body's digestive system, bloating, constipation and increased gases become your new normal.

In practice, this means you're going to need a new pair of jeans, your bathroom is about to become your favourite room in the house, and you will spend a good part of your day perfecting the art of silent farting.

Bloating diminishes after menopause…just joking!

WE NEED TO TALK ABOUT WEIGHT GAIN

To calculate a dog's age, there's a popular rule of thumb stating that *one dog year equals seven human years.*

The same rule applies for menopause pounds. (Or it should.)

1 pound lost during menopause is the equivalent of 7 pounds lost before your hormones decided to die.

Menopause pounds come (easily) and go (straight down to your midsection).

When oestrogen levels slow down, your metabolism (which processes energy) and your muscle production and repair functions slow down too.

This means that if you maintain the exact same activity level and eat the exact same amount of cookies that you did before menopause, the metabolic changes provoked by menopause will make you gain the exact number of pounds that you need to feel crappy.

But wait, there's more…

The shrinking in oestrogen levels also makes you more sensitive to carbohydrates, so the probability of that second plate of pasta being stored as fat instead of being burned right away as energy is not just a probability anymore.

Do you know the expression: 'Don't kick people when they're down?'

Well, menopause doesn't. Here's a little extra…

With age, muscle mass unsurprisingly drops for women (and men), but when women lose oestrogen (which is their main muscle-builder), the decline is more significant. Of course it is.

Muscles burn more energy than fat, so when the ratio of lean muscle mass to fat drops, it feeds back to the menopause-related drop in your metabolic rate.

The result? The new natural lifebuoy around your waist, AKA the menopause belly.

Yup, Toto, we're not in Kansas anymore!

BODY GLORY

I had been cohabiting with menopause for about a year when I detected that it was starting to take up more space in my life than we had initially agreed on.

Out of all the glitches that kept piling up on my menopausal inventory, my body's general functioning (or malfunctioning in this case) was what frustrated me the most.

Waking up as if I had come second place at the Ironman World Championship the day before became a monthly occurrence; throwing out my back from picking something up from the floor – like my dignity – became a justified phobia.

Little everyday injuries here and there that appeared without warning and for the lamest reasons began to multiply.

From leaving a Zumba class after ten minutes (the warm-up) to throw up in the bathroom because my heart was racing like a Formula 1 McLaren, to locking my knee while on the toilet during a lunch at my sister's in-laws – I learned to unlock it all by myself that day – I proudly began collecting injuries in the most awkward situations.

I also developed Achilles tendonitis on not one but both feet. With that sad blow, I realised that menopause didn't just take your looks, your sanity and your hormones; it took things you loved, too.

I used to be a jogger.

Let me rephrase that.

I used to be addicted to jogging. Every day, seven days a week, I would start my mornings with an 8km run.

Ah, the 'runner's high'... that euphoric state where the release of endorphins makes you feel like, if you took just one more step, you could actually fly. I experienced it every day.

Every day, I would run from my worries, from my problems, from the world. I found utter refuge in this form of exercise, which many find so boring.

With my double tendonitis, the simple act of walking became a daily agony – one that was with me for over three years.

After encountering a large assortment of doctors and therapies spread over those three years, I went to see yet another specialist who told me:

'For the tendonitis, take a rest from walking, ice it daily and see what happens. But look, N, as of now, with menopause, you need to accept the fact that your body is only going to function at 70% capacity.'

I looked him straight in the eye, making sure he could read the disapproval in mine, and confidently threw out an *I don't think so.*

And I was right. My body didn't function at 70%, as

the *mean* doctor so arrogantly suggested. In the years that followed, my body functioned at 62%, thank you very much!

As for my tendonitis, after months of resting – and walking as little as possible, like the doctor had advised me to – it got much better; but by that time other little menopausal booboos had developed, meaning I would never jog again.

O.S.T.E.O.P.E.R.O.S.I.S

Ostroperosis.

Osteperosis.

Wait… osteroporosis.

Let me try again… oestoperosis.

OK… Osteo-my-bones-are-givin'-me-a- flippin'-neurosis.

In an everlasting quest to have the last laugh at our expense, menopause didn't think it was bad enough to throw this bone deterioration dossier in our face – it had to be unpronounceable too.

But why?

Why the complicated, unsayable name? Where is its short and easy nickname counterpart?

Just like viral gastroenteritis is called a stomach bug, viral rhinitis is a cold and nuchal rigidity is known as a stiff neck – couldn't osteoporosis have a shortcut too?

Bonosis would be nice. It has 'bone' in it – which we've used most of our lives – and ends with 'osis', so those in the medical profession are happy and can feel important.

Bonosis could even trick our brains into thinking it was actually something good. (Like *bonuses*.)

'The results came back – you've got Bonosis.'

'Oh, how wonderful! Thank you, doctor.'

AND ARTHRITIS...

Unlike osteoporosis, where the bones become weaker and more likely to fracture, arthritis is a more complex disease that causes joint pain and reduces mobility and function. (But it is easier to pronounce... just saying.)

Although these two conditions have different causes and treatments, they can both cause pain around the bones and joints.

Which is less bad?

Well, pain is the main symptom of arthritis, and it affects specific joints... so let's start there.

Osteoporosis, on the other hand, is all fun and games until you break a bone. (Not to be confused with *breaking a leg*, which is supposed to bring luck; breaking a bone brings only pain. Lots of it.)

Also, the pain of a broken bone can be temporary... or chronic. (And something tells me that the chronic often wins!)

In the end, really... *all roads lead to Rome.*

Either you get there on crutches or with a brand-new tottering hip – that's entirely for Dame Menopause to decide.

BLADDER CONTROL TO MAJOR NONE

As the menopausal saga continues, here's another significant piece that will hang nicely on your f***-you-menopause-really-f***-you wall.

Bladder control.

Less elastic skin, weaker pelvic floor, hormones (or lack thereof) – you know the drill.

Now on top of not being able to control their nerves, some women may find it difficult to control their urinary flow.

On both fronts, they are pissed. (Pun intended – yes, I totally intended this one.)

And since good things come in threes, frequent urination and urge incontinence decided it was a good time to jump on the bladder bandwagon.

Now…

If you have a fragile bladder, there are four activities you may need to accomplish with the utmost care from this moment on: sneezing, coughing, lifting and – to my greatest dismay – laughing.

1. Sneezing

First of all, forget about 'you snooze, you lose'; your new-found motto is 'you sneeze, you squeeze.'

And you pray to God that you can hold it all in.

Squeezing your upper legs together as forcefully as if your life, your dignity and your underwear depended on it has proven to be quite efficient, if done with complete mental focus.

Crossing your legs, although more noticeable to bystanders, offers better chances of success.

It is crucial that the squeeze be performed before the sneeze occurs. This chronology is key; otherwise, any attempt will be as useless as putting a stop sign in the middle of a car crash scene.

2. Coughing

Same strategy applies with coughing. But while sneezing requires one big focus on the bladder control centre, coughing needs a little more emphasis and endurance, because you don't just cough once, right?

In that case, good control of the lungs can come in handy too. Holding back your cough or trying to limit the number of exhalations escaping from your throat can reduce the risk of unsolicited fluid escaping from your bladder. Strangely, the lungs and bladder seem to be working in tandem, which means you should hold your breath for as long as you humanly can.

Not to burst anyone's sac here, but if your bladder's

weakness magnitude scores six or more on the Outflow Scale using the common base ten logarithm, your case is close to hopeless.

You might as well go with the embarrassing flow.

3. Lifting

I strongly believe that after a certain age, lifting should be a concept a woman engages with on specific occasions only.

Examples:

I want a mini face-lift.

[While typing www.net-a-porter.com] I need to lift my mood.

I'll take the lift, of course.

Can you give me a lift home? I want to go home. Now.

Ideally, anything heavier should be lifted by some gracious, helpful *someone else*.

4. Laughing (sad-face emoji)

While laughter in general doesn't go well with a feeble bladder, a side-splitting laugh will take your pee pouch to a whole new leak zone where no amount of holding, squeezing, pressing and praying can save you.

It's called collateral damage, and it's OK.

When your laughter unexpectedly becomes uncontrollable, when you suddenly feel like you have cracked open the gates of endorphin city and a trancelike fit of giggles has begun to invade your system (bladder included), you shouldn't think twice.

You embrace the happy hormone party (hormones, everyone, hormones!) and accept the leakage casualty with an open bladder.

As a matter of fact, you carpe diem the life out of this moment because, let's face it, what's a little unsolicited organic fluid compared to a torrent of oxytocin, dopamine and endorphins?

Remember those?

At the peak of my menopause, I once followed my own advice above.

I held on to that exhilarating moment, as well as to a lamppost in Amsterdam. Legs squeezed and crossed, lower body stock-still, I desperately waited for my urge to laugh to become weaker than my urge to pee.

For three long minutes, surrounded by my party posse in hysterics too, I had to fight the impulse to pee and to laugh simultaneously.

Torn between which one I should surrender to, and clearly not encouraged by the pack of hyenas in stiches surrounding me, this proved to be one of the most excruciating exercises in willpower I had to face during my menopausal summit.

Miraculously, I did beat the odds that day. I had my blissful hormonal cake and ate it too – without making a mess.

I laughed to the point of tears, and got out of it with pants and dignity intact. (If you don't count the lamp post I hugged for three minutes.)

N: 1.

Menopause: 0.

PALPITATION NATION

There's a way the heart beats when you've just fallen in love and you're about to meet the object of your desire again.

An exhilarating countdown, where your heart delightfully loses control. It races, skips a beat, flutters and pounds, and you welcome all these cardiac irregularities with excitement and anticipation, because you know that soon you and your other half will be reunited in one big bubble of pleasure and bliss…

Oh, the elation, the delight, the sheer eagerness.

During the hormone-massacre rampage, you may experience heart fluttering, pounding, racing and skipping more than a beat too. Only you're not counting down the exhilarating minutes that will bring you to your new love, just the ones that will bring the water to boil so you can have your afternoon tea – which you don't really want anymore, because now you're busy speculating over whether you're having the preliminary stages of a heart attack or something like that.

These palpitations may feel the same as being in love, but no, they're not. You're not.

And I'm sorry, but if it looks like a duck, swims like a duck and quacks like a duck… it's not necessarily a duck. It could be menopause invading your cardiovascular system or wanting to finish off whatever is left of your paranoid state.

FATIGUE AND LAZINESS, POTATO POTAHTO

Why is it that when a woman says she's tired, the rest of the world often assumes she's just being lazy or whiny?

She could be a working single mother of three, running around from dusk till dawn, juggling snack boxes and annual company reports, but if she says 'I'm tired' she will still need to defend her fatigue with solid arguments before she gets any validation.

'I ran a marathon, then came back home, showered and made lasagna from scratch for the kids. I helped them with their homework, before writing a piece on the origins of octopus polygamy. I washed the car, I made myself a chamomile tea and went to bed. I was so tired'.

People will often retain 'chamomile' and 'tired', and raise their eyebrows in a *stop whining* kind of way.

The rest will try to top your fatigue with their own exhaustion.

'Oh yeah? Well, I ran a marathon, then came back home, showered and made lasagna from scratch for the kids. I helped them with their homework, before writing a piece on the origins of octopus polygamy. I washed the car too. Then I made myself a chamomile tea, PLUS did ten jumping jacks and THEN went to bed.'

Menopause fatigue is different.

Menopause fatigue doesn't require you to do jumping jacks or make lasagna to be tired, because your hormones are doing Ironman and preparing an Italian buffet in there. And while you're lying on the couch staring at a blank wall, seemingly doing absolutely nothing, your system is literally fighting for dear life, when it's not crumbling like the last days of Rome.

Oh and also, menopause doesn't serve chamomile tea.

An interesting fact about menopausal exhaustion is that very often it just crashes down on your day without warning, and within seconds, your energy levels go from pumping-up-the-jam to brain-dead.

The fatigue a woman feels during menopause is real, and it's pretty incapacitating. It grips your body, your energy, your soul, and most importantly your brain, or whatever cells are left of it.

Think of menopause fatigue as a gold-digger with whom you forgot to sign a pre-nup, because you never suspected it would try to take everything from you!

SIGHT AND SEEING AND BEING SEEN

As the menopausal army progresses on all fronts, some women may face vision alterations, which might require them to start wearing glasses – if they didn't already.

But as it turns out, wearing glasses does have its advantages…

Pros
Shopping for glasses is like shopping for heels used to be – back when you could still wear heels. There were so many ways to express your sensuality through these extra centimetres.

Red soles, porn-star heels, sexy stilettos, boots that weren't made for walking; when you shopped for sizzling shoes, there was a story you would inevitably buy along with them. Manolo, Jimmy and Christian were the golden trinity and for decades dictated the attitude and altitude of many women's feet.

Despair not.

Glasses will offer you the same glorious sensation.

Take some thick red-framed glasses out of your bag to read the text some borderline harassing online store sent you about their new promotion – a text which, by the way, you're getting daily because you don't know how to unsubscribe from their stupid mailing list – and watch people's reactions once you drop these scarlet specs on your nose.

One thing I have noticed is that with glasses, the bigger and bolder you go, the more admiration and *vavavoom* points you score.

OK, so we're not talking about the hot stilettos level of *vavavoom* that makes men want to take you home for a nightcap, but hey, all the better! We don't want to go home with anyone for a nightcap.

All we want is a little compliment here, a little validation there. A little 'Wow, darling, you audacious little thing, where did you get these from? I love the look,' and then we want to go home to our furry Birkenstocks and Isotoner slippers… and our comfortable nightcap-free sofa/bed/kitchen counter.

Glasses also make you look intellectual and/or important, which is the perfect way to conceal the inner pandemonium going on behind the scenes during menopause.

Cons
Well… your eyesight is sh*t now.

MENOLOOK

BAD HAIR DAY (CADE)

It's pretty fascinating to realise the extent to which, before menopause, our glorious hormones had been silently holding our mind, body and soul together all that time.

I shamefully assumed they were solely responsible for periods and babies, and I was never curious enough to even wonder about the vastness of their superpowers.

I took my hormones for granted.

I'm sorry, OK?

Skin, bones, sleep... it turns out that all along, hormones were actually caretakers for our health, with a firm 'never complain, never explain' stance.

I said I'm sorry!

Any declining aspect of a woman's physical and mental constitution that begins to take effect after menopause seems to be linked to her hormones (or lack thereof).

Joint pain? Hormones (or lack thereof).
Libido drop? Hormones (or lack thereof).
Mood swings? Hormones (or lack thereof).
Weight gain? Hormones (or lack thereof).

You name it, menopause seems to be on a mission to wreck it!

Hair tu, Brute?

Yup… hair too!

One of a woman's most prized and praised features is also part of the whopping menopausal everything-must-go stripdown!

But if losing one's mind because of menopause is one thing, losing one's hair is everything. Ask these women:

- Rapunzel
- Cleopatra
- Marilyn Monroe
- Farah Fawcett
- Audrey Hepburn
- Diana Ross
- Jackie Kennedy
- Princess Diana
- Anna Wintour

It wouldn't be an understatement to say that a woman's hair is one of her most treasured attributes. It's the blueprint of her looks, the organic signature she has personally created and chosen to represent her identity.

Throughout history, culture, religion and philosophy, a woman's hair has always been a reflection of her individuality and temperament, but also a projection of her era, her beauty, her fertility and femininity, her youth and grace…

The relationship between a woman's hair and her self-esteem is deeply rooted and deeply personal.

If we could measure a woman's brainwaves when she enters a hair salon sporting a scruffy greasy ponytail and then leaving it an hour later looking like the lion queen, I wouldn't be surprised if the neurological outcome equalled a good old Prozac pop downed with a fresh glass of Chardonnay on a Jamaican beach.

Unless Edward Scissorhands went on a coke binge before styling her hair, a woman will usually leave a hair salon acting like she's the newly appointed L'Oréal ambassador, and feeling like if anyone's worth it, it's her.

When a woman's hair looks glorious and gorgeous, she instantly feels glorious and gorgeous.

On the other hand, too dry, too frizzy, too thin, too unruly, and she is set for a grumpy ~~ponytail~~ day.

Knock knock…
Who's there?
Menopause.
Menopause who?
Meno-pause what's left of your enthusiasm – I'm here to wreck your hair too.

I'm not going to talk about the receding hairline that seems to be marching up our foreheads like an army of misogynistic hobgoblins.

I'm not going to talk about the upsetting hair thinning that prevents many women from wearing their hair long ever again for fear of looking like the creepy old lady in a white nightgown who slowly trails people in horror movies.

I'm not going to talk about that feeling of (hair) loss

you experience at every stroke of the brush, either. Too depressing.

And I'm certainly not going to talk about wigs and hair extensions and clip-ons, because I am a true believer in *whatever floats your boat*. If it helps, do it. Really, do it.

I'm going to talk about Bob and Pixie.

Not the genius musician/activist/*do-they-know-it's-Christmastime* Bob and his model/activist/singer daughter Pixie.

No, not the Geldof family.

I'm going to talk about the pixie and bob that concern us here.

The Louise Brooks hairdo/hair-rescue hotline/perfect hairstyle- pixie and bob cuts.

Because no matter how depressed our scalp may feel, the truth is, a woman sporting an elegant, immaculate and sophisticated hairdo with confidence will always win in the rock-paper-scissors game of hair.

So, sure, for many of us our good old days of Scarlett O'Hara hair are numbered, but let's be honest, our good hair days are not!

GLORIOUS GREY

The big grey hair dilemma.

Whoever came up with the *grey hair don't care* motto needs to be bitch-slapped.

Daily.

No matter how you put it, women *do* care about their hair colour, and last time I checked, to most people in our society, grey still meant old, it still meant scruffy and it still meant you literally didn't care about looking old and scruffy.

Ever since dyeing my grey roots became a monthly annoyance, I have been paying attention to the grey hair dialogue raging out there, and to the voices encouraging women like me to embrace their age and natural colour.

They're not grey hairs, they're wisdom highlights.
Every grey hair tells a story.
Grey hair is a crown of glory.
Stop it. Stop it now.
My age? I embrace. No problem.
My grey invasion? Well, here's a question.

Can you name five A-list actresses with grey hair, other than Halle Berry in X-Men?

Not that we need to follow the Hollywood agenda by any means, but I can count on one hand the number of women under fifty-five that have been part of my life – Hollywood and my own neck of the woods included.

I know one. I know her really well, actually.

It's my mother.

And when in her late forties she decided to embrace the silver-toned look, I cannot begin to describe the torrent of criticism and judgement (including mine) she had to face for simply accepting and welcoming Mother Nature's law.

Today I am older than she was when she decided to let time run its course, and even though I had a model of hair power and resilience right under my nose, I am still far too insecure and in denial to go Georgette Clooney any time soon.

I mean, I would really love to *not* go to the hairdresser every four weeks; I would love to avoid the damaging chemicals that are brushed onto my roots month after month. I would love to give my thinning, receding hair a *forever* break!

But it's too hard.

I tried.

And it really was too hard.

I felt self-conscious.

I felt scruffy.

I felt older.

I felt insecure.

I felt unkempt.

I also felt people looked at me differently… looked down on me a little.

I felt discomfort about the comments from some.

I felt exactly the way society expected me to feel.

I managed to go as far as two centimetres of grey roots before running back to my hairdresser like a pigment junkie and begging him to lay the damaging stuff on my roots again.

And when he did, I left the hair salon feeling relieved and neat and me again.

Not L'Oréal-ambassador good, but good enough to be OK with what I saw in the mirror.

Despite my belief in women's power and 'you go girl' attitude, grey equalling old and/or scruffy has been ingrained in my brain for so long that it has become my truth.

I wish I hadn't been brainwashed into associating silver-hued female hair with a sense of lack or ending, but I am not quite ready to change my mindset or my hair colour yet.

And it seems that neither is the world:

'Synonyms of *old*: *grey-haired* and/or *grey*.'

And right there, I rest my dyed hair's case.

THE SILVER FOX THEORY

And now, ladies and gentlemen, we will be taking a brief intermission prior to the rest of menopause's ravages to discuss George Clooney's – and his buddies' – silvery audacity.

I recently discovered that the male celebrities that rocked my childhood (Anderson Cooper, Hugh Grant, Patrick Dempsey) are flaunting their Silverado hair with such pride, and the media is sucking up to them with such fervour, that some millennials are actually going grey before their time just to look like them!

While we women are having gallons of ammonia and oxidising agents poured over our sorry heads monthly, surprise, surprise: greying men are now considered buzzworthy.

'Life is unfair, get used to it,' said another famous grey-haired man.

Well, let me tell you this…

The only reason we celebrate men's grey hair is because many of us have daddy issues and it gives us a sense of security and safety. Subconsciously, it makes us believe that we're in the presence of a great caretaker with experience and wisdom.

In fact, according to some deeply serious studies, it has very little to do with a man's hotness, sensuality or dashing looks.

So. Now. Can we please, once and for all, put the *Fifty Shades of Grey* nonsensical rubbish to rest? Thank you.

TEN (MENOPAUSAL) BEAUTY FACTS!

1. Your lips become thinner. Now would be a good time to look for new ways to express annoyance or sexiness, other than the traditional pout.
2. Your eyebrows also get thinner. (Look up: Benefit Cosmetics 24-Hour Brow Setter Clear Brow Gel with Lamination Effect.)
3. The hair on your scalp migrates to your face, because where else would it go?
4. Nails can become brittle and develop vertical ridges. Remember your nasty old maths teacher's nails when she used to point at the blackboard while yelling in your face?
5. Your smile lines become a permanent fixture. Nothing to smile about here – it means your cheeks are saggy all the time now.
6. Teeth can experience discoloration, and may appear yellowish… Say ~~CHEESE~~ MENOPAUSE!

7. Little brown spots and patches may appear on your face. They are darker than your skin tone, because if they were the same colour, nobody would notice.
8. Your eyelashes' growth slows down – to match that of your eyebrows. And your hair.
9. Rosacea. R.O.S.A.C.E.A.
10. RDF (Resting Droopy Face) is your new RBF (Resting Bitch Face).

CHIN CHIN

As we covered previously, the menopause facial hair offensive is real; it's not in your head.

Actually, it's mainly on your chin.

You first start developing a little duvet of hairs on your sideburn areas. Usually, these are quite subtle and even; most of the time they are only discernible if someone is looking at you through a magnifying glass.

The chin part is trickier.

Do you remember that game we used to play as kids – whack-a-mole? Mole heads would pop out of holes in the ground and you had to pound them with a plastic hammer. The more you pounded, the faster other mole heads would randomly emerge.

If you do remember, I hope you've kept the skills you used back then, because your chin is the ground now, and instead of the hammer, you're granted tweezers and a magnifying mirror.

The principle remains the same, but instead of pushing mole heads down, you have to pluck nasty hairs out.

Every time a hair pops out on your chin, you have to pluck it as fast as possible. It is necessary that you remain alert, because they appear in the most arbitrary ways, just like the moles did forty years ago.

The tweezer game, however, comes with a slight variation. While as a kid, when you were tired of whacking moles, you could just turn the whole thing off and move on to the next distraction, the tweezer game has no off switch, and there are no other distractions more important than keeping your chin a hair-free zone.

PIMP MY WARDROBE

A friend of mine once told me that the secret to looking amazing during menopause is *to look like sh*t most of the time*. 'Then, the minute you do your hair, add a little lipstick here and a pair of sexy heels there, people are instantly amazed.'

I personally find it very easy to look like sh*t during menopause, without even having an agenda.

I just dress according to my mood, and very often my mood calls for a hasty ponytail, a comfortable top and my favourite pair of jeans.

Make-up means drawing a line on top of my new Jean Harlow eyebrows and applying a touch of glossy tinted lip balm that will dissolve before I even make it to my front door.

Oh, and trainers… I'm never without my trainers. (You know… tendonitis and all.)

I must confess, laziness and a profound lack of motivation became my menopausal style.

After decades of hibernation, my inner rebel suddenly

woke up just to scream: 'I'm done making an effort with my looks – who's looking anymore, anyway? I'm fifty!'

My inner rebel has always been an idiot.

Let's be fair – wardrobe-wise, we are a lucky generation of menopausal peeps.

When my mother was my age, wearing trainers or a jazzy sweater, or even jeans, was a luxury you simply couldn't afford unless your name was Jane Birkin, Stevie Nicks or Tina Turner.

Back in the eighties, a woman's style after a certain age was bound to rigid new guidelines, as if the House of Windsor was setting the rules for her wardrobe.

The style was unquestionably elegant, but totally lacking on the fun and cool front.

Big coats, tightly tailored clothes, big belts, big heels, big sunglasses, immaculate hair, loud perfume – entering your fifties was a far from comfortable affair.

Thankfully, things have changed and today there's nothing absurd or scandalous about a woman sporting trendy trainers and a good pair of jeans whether she's in her fifties, sixties, seventies or even eighties.

You can be of a certain age and wear a casual style without the world assuming you're a sad individual hanging on to her youth, or a fashion victim.

Most importantly, you don't have to change your entire wardrobe to adapt to this new chapter of your life.

You can keep your jeans (if they still fit), your sexy tops (if they make you feel sexy), your miniskirts (if you still have the courage to wear them); you can keep your sneakers, and you can keep on feeling free to wear whatever makes you happy.

There are, however, some adjustments that can be made if you want to maximise your comfort.

1. Russian doll layering
   Given that during menopause a woman's bodily thermostat doesn't care if she's in the middle of a desert or locked inside a freezer, mastering the art of layering is more than a necessity – it's an obligation. You need to be able to strip off as easily and as fast as if Kevin Costner were in bed waiting for you, and you were actually in the mood for Kevin Costner waiting for you in bed.

2. Cotton is the new black
   It's one of the few fabrics that absorb humidity, sweat and embarrassment, and it also conducts heat – from your body to somewhere over the rainbow. 100% cotton is the Nelson Mandela of hot flash negotiators.

3. Go loose or go home
   Tight clothes can sometimes feel like a suffocating second skin, especially if and when hot flashes occur. So, remember:
   Better loose than sorry.

4. Camouflage me softly
   Think of army prints, but for social occasions like a loud cocktail party or a mandatory boring dinner party. The purpose of camouflage prints here is not to overpower your adversary, but your hot flashes. We want to deceive people into believing that we are absolutely not dripping our life away under that crisp, fresh floral top.

5. Cool and comfortable: your new comfort zone
   These two adjectives should be the new pillars of your wardrobe.

   Every time you are about to acquire a new piece of clothing, try it on and repeat ten times, very quickly: 'I'm sweating like an old cow in a slaughterhouse.'

   Hopefully it will help you decide whether the piece makes the cut.

MENOLIFE

ALL THE MENOPAUSAL LADIES... PUT A LID ON IT!

When you're in your twenties, love is impulsive, unreasonable, all-consuming and, more often than not, downright reckless.

'You feel like nobody gets you? Me too… we're so similar! I love you. We're soulmates, you and me; it's forever, it's beyond belief, it's us against the universe, let's go to Thailand and watch the sunset together, let's change the world…'

Oh, the sweetness of being in love at twenty.

Desire is your main radar, and it uses your libido-waves to determine the distance and radial velocity between you and your next orgasm.

You are young, beautiful and hopeful – and so are your hormones. Biology is on your side, too, with your drive to reproduce in full force.

Falling in love, being in love, drowning in love; you only need to watch one episode of a reality TV show to understand how far hormones will take you when you're in your twenties, how many times they'll take you there, and with how many partners.

Love in your twenties feels like an eternal dance, a beginning with no end. It feels like you have found the reason you were born.

You. Were. Born. To. Love.

At fifty, you have found the *real* reason why you were born.

You were born to love – sure, whatever – but mainly you were born to decipher the intricate manual of this crazy thing called life.

You were also born to suffer *just a little* in the process.

From Gandhi to Socrates to Dumbo the elephant, the *life is suffering* dogma is hard to miss.

Jingle hell, jingle hell, red flags all the way!

And yet when you're in your twenties and in love, you manage to miss them all, over and over again.

At fifty, however, you just can't miss the red flags anymore. You don't want to miss them. You won't miss them.

Destiny has taken a gigantic poop on your love boat – a few times, too – and now, before you decide to embark on an impulsive romantic voyage, you list the pros and cons, you call your therapist and your gynaecologist, you check with your astrologer, you watch an episode of *True Crime* on Netflix, and you sleep on it.

It's called wisdom.

So, if and when you happen to fall for someone in a way that bears some resemblance to falling in love, you do not jump straight in.

You use your menopausal brain cells instead of letting your foolish heart spontaneously lead the way.

You're wise now, remember?

First you ask yourself: 'What's in it for me?' Because you're proficiently pragmatic now; you've seen the movies, read the books, lost the one that got away, been there, done that, believed, been dumped, been cheated on, sobbed, found the light, been reborn from the ashes – twice over – and reached the humble conclusion that *Il vaut mieux être seul que mal accompagné* (it's better to be alone than in bad company).

Only this time you really mean it, because you know it's true.

Then you ask yourself: what is love without libido or the need to procreate? What is love if you're emotionally independent? What is love if you no longer have the energy for an exchange of sob stories and traumas? What is love if you don't want to be someone's mother, maid, therapist, punching bag?

Love is like an iPhone update bringing new, fun and valuable features. It's being with someone who will bring your existing levels of happiness and peace (the levels you fought for a lifetime to attain) from a solid 85% to 95%. That's what love is.

And to get there, well, you scan your new love interest. And you scan them good.

- What's their opinion on the occasional hot dog?
- What time do they usually wake up?
- Are they team *Friends* or team *Seinfeld*?
- If you're at a party and want to leave early, what do they do? (Be careful, that's a trick question.)
- What music do they listen to in the car? What about the volume?

- If they ask you 'What's wrong?' and you answer 'Nothing,' what do they do?
- What's their opinion on climate change?
- What's their health situation?
- Any allergies to pets?
- How many Covid jabs did they get?
- What's their opinion on partners having separate bedrooms?
- What's their ex's number, so you can fact-check their answers?

Once they successfully pass this first test, it's on to phase two: probation period.

The probation period is one that requires you to be at your most alert and focused, because after all these years you know better than you used to, and you recognise that it's all in the details.

The way they animatedly gesture with their hand while holding their fork might be cute today, but a year from now, it will be the exact reason you stab them with that very same fork.

So you notice things. You take note.

They cancel plans last-minute with a lame excuse?

You take note. They're unreliable.

They're on their phone browsing Facebook during a dinner date?

You take note. They're ill-mannered.

They badmouth their ex-girlfriend/ex-wife and share her deepest secrets?

You take note. They're untrustworthy.

They're rude to the waiter?

You take note. They're a douche.

No confrontation needed here. Who can be bothered to have an argument with someone who just tore the poor waiter to shreds because their food came forty-five seconds later than yours?

No conflict needed, either. You silently take note, and then you assess.

If you find the perfect partner *you haven't been looking for*, then you jump in and thank your lucky stars for sending such a like-minded, decent human being your way.

You can walk through this next chapter of your life with a plus one.

If, on the other hand, the person doesn't meet your criteria, then you dispose of them. No explanation needed, no 'It's not you, it's me' (it's probably THEM!), no regrets, no justification – you simply dispose of them.

And you know why?

Because *that's showbiz, baby*!

KAMA SUTRA LIMITED

Unless you're the actual lovechild of Linda Lovelace and Benjamin Button, there's a big chance that with menopause:

1. You can't cover 93% of the Kama Sutra anymore.
2. You're not remotely interested in covering even 3.99% of it.

Your kids are all grown up now, you have more time on your hands than you need, no more periods, no risk of getting pregnant – but oh, sweet irony, no oestrogen either, and consequently no desire.

You get more pleasure and anticipation from watching Ina Garten prepare grilled cheese sandwiches and lemonade for her friends Tyler and Michael, waiting to get their pictures taken in the garden, than from season 1, episode 3 of Sex/Life on Netflix. (Yes, episode 3.)

Menopause is to sex what gastritis is to a free Michelin-starred meal.

You would love to have it if only your body weren't so busy dealing with more urgent matters.

Your new sex toys now come in tubes and boxes and bottles and pills: lubricants, suppositories, vaginal moisturisers and prescription drugs with names like AH!YES and Candid-CL and Gynella... because, let's face it, your crazy, slutty libido has left the building. For good.

What you have instead is a vaginal desert, an intense lack of desire, recurring hip pain, doubts and insecurities about this new body of yours that suddenly seems to understand the laws of gravity, distinctly decreased stamina, and perhaps also a partner going through his own age-related alterations, who may be needing the help of a little blue pill to get the party going.

'Do you want have sex?'

'No.'

'Yeah, me neither. Let me take a Viagra, then.'

'OK.'

'Ready?'

'No.'

'Me neither, let's do it!'

'Yup, let's do it!'

Regarding the Barefoot Contessa's grilled cheese sandwiches, either cheddar or Gruyère works fine... I checked.

SEX AND THE PITY

In 1979, former US vice president and prominent member of America's wealthiest family Nelson Rockefeller died of a heart attack while having sexual intercourse with Megan Marshack, his twenty-five-year-old assistant.

He was seventy.

I am not sure if this qualifies as a happy ending, but it certainly raises awareness of the hazards of sex past a certain age.

Let's face it – if, after menopause, the mere act of sleeping can spark injuries (think stiff neck and lower back pain), it is safe to say that sex is now a booby-trapped territory holding a portfolio of minor and major liabilities.

Less endurance, less pleasure, less flexibility, less libido… more 'Wait,' 'Are you OK?' 'Ouch, my knee,' and 'Hold on… my back…'

As menopause progresses, sex becomes a series of stop-start interludes where you manage to slip in a few ooohhhhs, ahhhhs and ohhhhs here and there.

Despite what some media and prescription drug

adverts would have us believe, intercourse in later years isn't as pleasurable for most men and women as it used to be; nor is it as frequent as they'd like us to think.

As you age, blood fills your genitals more slowly when you become aroused, which means you don't have the same sensitivity anymore and reaching orgasm takes longer, if it's ever reached at all.

When getting aroused or having an orgasm becomes a time-consuming challenge with a milder reward than the one we've been used to getting for most of our life, it's only logical that we become discouraged and reticent.

I mean, would you participate in a competition and put in the same effort if the winning prize was a plastic sushi maker, after decades of feasting at Nobu?

Add to that the sexual pharmaceuticals some have to rely on for a sub-microscopic orgasm, and it won't be difficult to understand why your sex life has officially gone fishing.

The equation is simple:

Vaginal dryness + erectile dysfunction = movie & pizza.

And quite frankly, that's arousing enough for me.

TIT FOR TAT

Don't drink and drive.

Also.

Don't eat and sleep.

'I will start with the tomatoes and mozzarella, please, then I'll have the filet mignon with mushroom sauce, and grilled vegetables and a baked potato on the side.'

'A little house red wine, maybe? Shall we share a bottle?'

'Oh, we need to order in advance for the chocolate fondant? Shall we share? OK then, four chocolate fondants it is. I just love chocolate fondant with my espresso.'

This is a recurrent 9pm conversation my friends and I would reliably have when going out for dinner. The menu would vary, of course, but the calorific content, the alcohol, the caffeine and the sugar wouldn't. Back then we hardly ever suffered from late-night dining, because our digestive systems were functional machines, silently performing ingestion, propulsion, digestion and absorption while we were busy LIVING LIFE.

Ignorance was bliss, and so were these inconsequential suppers.

(I love the word supper… it instantly makes it an elegant poetic affair, no matter what you're eating. 'Let's order a triple burger with cheese for supper, shall we?')

The icing on the cake? (Pun intended again – yes, I love puns.)

Following these generous meals, we would go home and while our digestive systems did the night-shift crackdown (or so we thought), we slumbered for the next nine plus hours.

We slept so deeply, so intensely, that no amount of sun rays, neighbours' high-decibel hoovering or pet saliva could wake us up in the morning.

We slept.

A very good friend of mine said that when you start weighing up the pros and cons before ordering a sloppy burger after 7pm, you know you're officially *not young anymore*.

So we stop eating at 7pm.

We dine on soup or light fish, and a tiny piece of bread and cheese if we're feeling naughty.

We avoid caffeine and chocolate desserts, obviously.

We pay attention to quantity and size.

And still… there is a small probability that we might experience nocturnal heartburn, bloating and indigestion.

That's why I will always order the sloppy burger after 7pm if the burger is worth it and I really want it.

For Gaviscon is my witness, I will never choose wisdom over a good burger.

Or pizza.

Or chocolate fondant, too. I love chocolate fondant.
And a little espresso… for digestion!

MENO-MENU

STARTERS
Omega 3 titbits
Calcium casserole
DHEA bites
St John's wort with ginseng sprouts
Vitamin D Parma ham

MAIN COURSE (from our HRT garden)
Patches with a side of vaginal cream
Oestrogen gel served with good intentions
Tablets on a bed of hope
Mixed feelings (to share)

DESSERTS
Medley of antidepressants
No-bake(d) CBD platter
Sweet mindfulness

CHEF'S SPECIAL
Ask the chef for our hormone-free menu

ALCOHOL YOU IN A WEEK

Between the significant physical, mental and emotional upheaval a woman goes though during menopause, surely a nice little glass of wine comes in handy every now and then?

Well, it doesn't.

It comes with a price.

As she ages, a woman's body loses water volume. She is therefore less able to dilute alcohol in her system, which makes her that much more vulnerable to its effects.

In other words, *if you can't take the pain, don't play the game.*

I can still remember a time when my friends I and would hop from one party to another, from bar to disco, downing drinks and having fun until the morning light with such an invigorating sense of entitlement and frivolity.

We would dance for hours as if the whole world was watching – and we couldn't care less if it was – and then head to the shadiest joint – the only one that would still be open at 5am – to gulp down a delicious sandwich dripping with cholesterol, diabetes and salmonella.

Thirty minutes later, we would crash and sleep like babies for the next twelve hours.

Our bodies were hot, resilient instruments governed by our reckless minds. Bliss.

Alcohol was not something we sipped like *bon vivants*; it was something we downed like idiots. And boy was it fun!

It's not that we didn't care about its effect on our liver and our brain cells. We didn't even know we *had* livers or brain cells.

Eventually, with age and a serious expansion of our responsibilities (mortgages, babies, laundry), this electrifying era would make room for a calmer one, where drinking would become a less sloppy affair.

Rum and Cokes were gradually converted into Saint-Émilion and Grand Marnier; chaotic nights became grown-up dinners; and mild warning signals from our livers and brain cells started to flicker.

Regardless of these whopping changes, alcohol was still very much on our side.

Fast-forward a few decades – school plays, business trips, loss of a parent, empty nest, divorce, menopause...

And suddenly: poof!

Your liver and brain cells decide it's payback time!

Like, right now.

Drinking has now become a conditional indulgence with a bunch of nasty little impending punishments.

1. Drinking alcohol can trigger hot flashes. (Like super-hot hot flashes.)
2. Drinking alcohol can turn your cheeks bright red; not the you-*look-great-were-you-in-St-Moritz?* kind of red, more like Heidi's grandmother red.
3. Drinking alcohol increases wrinkles. (Of course it does.)
4. Drinking alcohol can affect your sleep. (Because it's not ruined enough yet.)
5. Drinking alcohol can cause depression – in case you're not sufficiently miserable already.
6. Drinking alcohol can cause hangover symptoms that may stay with you for up to a week. 7 days. 168 hours. Hangover.

It all comes down to two options.

Team Virgin Mary or team Bloody Mary.

Some women will plan for their next drink as if they are moving to a foreign country. *What's the occasion? What's my mood like today? What's on the menu? Who will be there? What time does it start?*

And if the game is worth it, they will endure the pain.

Others will just play the game, endure the pain and do it again and again!

SO I THOUGHT I COULD DANCE

Here's a little mystery.

What happens to our groove with age and time?

Do we lose it in one go while we're not paying attention, or does it progressively fade away, silently twirling on to the next generation?

I used to think I was quite a good dancer. Groove, moves, the whole party bundle; I genuinely believed I was one of the cool ones on the dance floor and in front of the mirror at home.

But then one day, my kids gave me the Elaine Benes from Seinfeld 'Little Kicks' reality check.

It seems I had either lost my once self-proclaimed legendary groove, or I never actually had one to start with.

Grindelwald, Switzerland, circa 1984. I am in the ballroom of a small resort, celebrating the New Year with my family.

I am thirteen. I think I own the world and the world

owes me everything. I think nobody gets me, but I get it. All of it!

And the universe is laughing. SO HARD.

My parents are laughing too. They are on the dance floor having the time of their life, and I am watching them as they boogie the night away. My heart is filled with pride and tenderness and love for them.

Still, I can't help but notice how clumsy their moves are – how, despite the incredible fun they seem to be having, they totally lack rhythm and beat.

Their moves combine remnants of the twist with a little disco and all the trendy dances they encountered in between.

Meanwhile, I am obsessed with *Footloose* and holding out for a hero named Kevin Bacon.

When I dance, I feel the same rage and passion he does in that epic warehouse scene. I feel THAT cool, too. (I'm sure you can picture the dynamic choreography taking place in our garage.)

So when I look at my parents and all their buddies on this vibrant Swiss dance floor, I have this overconfident sense of judgement tickling me.

Obviously, it doesn't tickle anymore.

As a matter of fact, it probably tickles my kids now, because today, I am *my parents dancing* and then some.

I have become so uncoordinated that even trying to memorise a ten-second TikTok dance is a challenge for me. (Yes, yes, I've tried with my nieces… and without.)

I have become so unbalanced that a single spontaneous movement now holds the possibility of a week on Voltaren.

And I have become so clumsy that I'm no longer holding out for a hero but for a chair most of the time.

Paradoxically, I have much more fun dancing today than I ever had in that warehouse with Kevin Bacon.

And it seems I am not alone. Most women of my generation appear to share that very same enthusiasm and dynamism when it comes to the relationship between ageing and dancing.

Recently, at a wedding, I noticed that most of my friends had adopted similar uncoordinated, unbalanced, ungraceful dance moves to mine, combined with an unapologetic sense of fun.

And the scene shot me right back to 1984.

This time, however, I could feel Mum and Dad's jubilant energy – electric, authentic, joyful and uninhibited. This time I felt like I was dancing with them.

And in a beautiful circle-of-life way, I really think I was.

So maybe I did once have a groove after all (or maybe not), and maybe time took it away, but one thing is for sure: it didn't take the fun.

All together now…

MENOMIND

MOOD SWING AND TWIST

You know how it goes.

You wake up in the best of moods.

If Alice in Wonderland had grown old enough, she would be you and you would be her.

You smile for no reason; you grab your pet in the hallway and imagine he understands you mumbling:

'Good morning, you – the best kitty-catto in the whole wide world.'

It doesn't matter that kitty-catto wants to scratch your face off and run under the bed.

You. Are. Blissful.

You even greet menopause with a little curtsy, thinking *let's be friends*, because why not? Life is good, you feel good – you want to sing it and share it with the birds, the trees, your slippers and the bathroom.

By the time you walk into the kitchen to make your first cup of coffee, though, just like in an incoherent bad dream, you feel you have suddenly stepped into *Apocalypse Now*!

Reason? Unknown.

But it's happening and it's real.

Life is sh*t, menopause is sh*t, your slippers are sh*t, your face is sh*t and everybody else's face is sh*t too. You're just angry, incensed, for no reason whatsoever, and you have this deep compulsion to smash something, anything, against the wall – like your boss' face or your coffee mug.

But just as you grab your cute little mug with kitty-catto's face on it, a shift takes place, and suddenly you are stricken with deep sadness and melancholy.

Oh, you precious little mug, oh, my poor little kitty-catto (still under the bed waiting for Mummy to be done being crazy) – and to think I was going to smash you...

Tears start rolling down your face, and before you know it, you are sitting on the kitchen floor, dramatically sobbing your heart out.

Oh dear God, whyyy? Why me? Why must I feel this pain? Life is too hard. I can't... I just can't anymore...

Reason? Still unknown.

But it's happening and it's real.

And then it stops. Out of nowhere. You're just done. You get up, wipe your nose and eyes, and place the coffee filter in the coffee basket before adding a big tablespoon of Lavazza to it as if nothing just happened.

Kitty-catto reappears: *Done yet, you lunatic b*tch? Can you freakin' feed me now?*

Menopause mood swings are completely out of the jurisdiction of logic. They're out of your control, too. They just happen, and all you can do is follow the dysfunctional trail of emotions through a random ride that will hopefully bring you back to your senses once it's done with you.

Who chooses to cry hysterically in the middle of a train station because they missed their train – when the next one is in fifteen minutes?

Who likes to make a hasty exit from the middle of the cinema queue because she feels like all the air has been sucked out of the planet?

Who yells at her drawer and then cries because it won't close properly?

Someone has taken the driver's seat, and it's now *Driving Miss Crazy*.

Reason? Still unknown.

But it's happening and it's real.

NEWTON'S GRAVE THEORY

Who hasn't heard the legendary story?

A young Isaac Newton is sitting under an apple tree when suddenly an apple falls on his head. In one of the biggest Eureka moments in the history of Eureka moments, he discovers that the same force that brought the apple to the ground also attracted the moon to the earth and the earth to the sun. Gravity.

It seems that for the first few decades of her life, a woman's face, breasts, buttocks and skin don't quite understand gravitational theory, and somehow it doesn't seem to apply to them either. A real win-win.

Her attributes remain perky, lifted and flexed; the only Newton she identifies with is Olivia. (Newton John.)

But then apples start raining on her head, and suddenly her body and mind remember to crash to the ground, Isaac Newton style.

To be fair, I was blessed with a baby face and a good set of genes, which helped me put off this *grave* moment until I was fifty-one.

Before menopause, people often thought I was almost a decade younger than my actual age. Guess-my-age used to be my one of my favourite games, and obviously one hell of an ego-booster – yes, I was vain and insecure like that.

Little by little, though, the guessing game became a no-fun charade where people would almost always actually guess my age.

'You're forty-nine?'

'Sure, whatever.'

I began inspecting my face with a combination of trepidation and fascination.

My cheeks, I think, were the part of my appearance I wasted the most time on. Every day I would see them drop, slump and fall a little further… I didn't like it. I didn't like it because they reminded me of my grandmother's cheeks, and although I loved my grandmother dearly, God bless her beautiful soul, I was not ready to be my grandmother quite yet. I wasn't even ready to be my mother, for what it's worth!

I wasn't upset about the new identity emerging on my face.

Sometimes I would recognise myself and sometimes I wouldn't, and that's normal and that's OK.

It was a little like when my boys were growing up and every now and then, they would walk into the room looking so much bigger than the minute before, and I would proudly say, 'Oh my, when did *that* happen?'

Every now and then, I would look at my face in the mirror and I too would perplexedly say, 'Oh sh*t, when did *that* happen?'

What I came to realise very soon, though, was that I genuinely didn't mind the wrinkles, the sagginess, the flabbiness of my face, hands, stomach and arms... I really didn't mind that the story of my life was distinctly mapped on my body and on my face, as if a hyper-ambidextrous person had traced it there.

It was the countdown I saw in it that troubled me sometimes.

My mortality.

TOLERANCE

Did you know that the word *tolerance* comes from the Latin terms *tolerare* and *tolerantia*, which suggest enduring, suffering, bearing, and forbearance?

Me neither, until I ran out of it.

I always considered myself a tolerant person.

You can identify as a carrot if it makes you happy, and I will respect you and accept it. I will respect you no matter what. As long as your choices don't step on mine...

One person's freedom ends where another's begins.

But I am not talking about that type of *tolerantia* here. Not religious, spiritual, racial or gender tolerance.

I am talking about the 'turn the other cheek' kind: the kind that involves sacrifice and patience; the kind that cooks an elaborate dinner and gets 'I don't like beef bourguignon. Can we order pizza?' when it's time to eat.

The tolerance that involves silent frustration and irritation; the kind that doesn't get *thank you*s; the kind that takes you for granted – and for a ride – simply because it can.

The kind that fortunately menopause has snatched from me.

So sure, I will turn the other cheek, but only for my head to take a good swing so I can headbutt you better.

We can blame this newly found intolerance on hormones and menopause all we want, but I personally find it quite liberating.

At fifty-one, it was high time to end my *tolerantias*, suffering, bearing, and forbearance.

BRAIN-FOG THIS SH*T!

Names below have been changed to protect the anonymity of victims of menopausal brain fog. Not that any of us will remember anyway... Oh wait, I'm not naming anyone!

Ten real-life brain fog situations:

1. You call your pet by your kid's name (or vice-versa) repeatedly and wonder why he's not answering.
2. You can name all the movies your favourite actress has been in without being able to remember her name... Oh... right... Cate Blanchett! (I love you, Cate Blanchett!)
3. You realise that for the past five minutes you have not listened to a single word your companion has said and you have absolutely no idea what the exchange was about. Incidentally, you wonder how on earth he/she didn't notice, since it was a one on one conversation.
4. You arrive at the supermarket and realise you've

left your grocery list at home. You drive back home and forget why you drove back home. You drive back to the supermarket – without the list.
5. You dial someone's number and by the time they answer, say 'Hello? Yes, who is this?'
6. You put your car keys in the fridge/the bathroom cupboard/your pocket/the cat's bed, and while pointing at the silver bowl on the table in the hall, you yell at your entire family, 'I'M NOT CRAZY! I SWEAR TO GOD, I PUT THEM RIGHT HERE!'
7. You count your supplements because you can't remember if you took your pill ten seconds ago.
8. You tell your child to turn down the music in the car so you can focus on the road.
9. So, it's the story of man who tells his wife to… oh no, sorry, the wife tells her husband that… err, no, no, it's a married couple talking and… forget it, I can't remember, but it's a really funny joke.
10. 9am: Good morning, Lydia, how are you?
10.30am: Good morning, Lydia, how are you?
Why is Lydia acting so weird today?
11am: Hello, Lydia, how are you today?

I CRY WITH MY LITTLE EYE

Menopausal tears are tricky. Kind of cruel, too.

They don't warn you if or when they will appear; they don't need an invitation or a valid reason. They just unexpectedly surface in your eye sockets, the same way a hot flash would on your face.

Just like a snooping neighbour or an inconsiderate mother-in-law, menopausal tears are uncontrollable and more often than not a little psychotic.

If you're lucky, they will just last a few seconds. Your eyes will experience a little sparkle before you can quickly recompose yourself. The tears are gone; your ego is safe.

If you are not so fortunate, they will stay around a little longer, and you will find yourself sobbing as if you were watching Susan Sarandon's final scene in *Stepmom* for the first time.

Menopausal tears flourish on certain dynamics.

They don't care if you're in a meeting, walking your dog or having lunch with your sister in a cool restaurant; as a matter of fact, they love appearing at the worst time.

You know… to add a humiliation factor to your sudden vulnerability.

Exhibitionist to the core, these tears enjoy supermarkets, elevators, cafés and meeting rooms. They bloom at contact with strangers and believe that crying in private is not half as fun as losing your sh*t in public.

Once they are over and you have exposed your fragile, defenceless side to the world, once your nose and eyes are red and your face puffed up enough, their job is done.

Merci… Until next time!

TEAR CONCENTRATION BAROMETER

- Talking about the past – 50%
- Feeling exhausted – 80%
- Missing your bus – 77%
- Not fitting into your jeans – 55%
- Family validation – 79%
- Bad night's sleep – 45%
- Your boss saying you did a bad job – 65%
- Your boss saying you did a good job – 65%
- Your boss – 65%
- *Only Love Can Hurt Like This* by Paloma Faith – 70%
- Someone asking 'Are you OK?' and meaning it – 55%
- Losing your phone – 65%
- Finding your phone – 89%
- TikTok about a dog adoption – 100%
- TikTok about a cat defending its babies – 100%

- TikTok about a friendship between a cow and a dog – 100%
- TikTok about two panda friends being separated – 100%
- TikTok about a gazelle sacrificing herself to save her baby from being devoured by a lion – 100%
- TikTok about a friendship between a dolphin and a cat – 100%

DEPRESSION, ANXIETY AND PANIC ATTACKS

When Dr S diagnosed me with early menopause, some of the questions that seemed most important to him, and which he insisted I answer pragmatically, were related to my mood.

'Do you feel like you're going crazy at times, N?' he candidly asked me.

Let's go into detail…
Mood swings?
Anxiety?
Panic attacks?
Depression?

When I officially menopaused, the man who would eventually become my ex-husband had just proposed, signalling the beginning of an all-consuming marriage.

At the time, I was also a functioning bulimic and had been for years on end – with all the emotional costs that entails.

These factors obviously contributed to blurring the lines around the real source of my anxiety and mood swings during menopause.

Bulimia? Menopause? Draining marriage? Life as we know it?

Who knows…

Let's just say that when menopause materialised in my head, it was already a very crowded place.

And so I surfed its psychological waves with a non-accusatory mindset, just going with the flow, without asking myself whose fault it was.

It just was.

If anything, I would soon realise that menopause ironically saved me.

MENO-SILVER LINING

GRASPING THE SILVER LINING

As women timidly cross the fifth-decade bridge of time, there comes a moment when some are confronted with an insistent echo, the sound of a long-lost self, repeating:

If not now, when?

A dream that remained just that, a dream.

The memory of a past love wrapped up in *what-ifs*.

An aspiration that is taking its last breaths.

A deep-rooted doubt that is suddenly burgeoning.

Is that it? Is it too late?

The unequivocal answer is no.

No, that is not it, and no, it's not too late, but only if you decide it's not.

LA DOLCE VITA

Anni, amori e bicchieri *di vino non si contano mai*
(Years, lovers and glasses of wine must never be counted)

I've always believed that Italians celebrate life more profoundly, sincerely and devotedly than anybody else in the world.

The happiness you will find in a modest *spaghetti aglio e olio*, a Lucio Battisti ballad or a drive in Val d'Orcia is difficult to replicate.

I was in my mid-twenties when I witnessed a captivating scene that would ricochet through my life decades later.

A quintessentially Italian story – *sì, certo!*

On the terrace of a Roman osteria, three ladies who seemed to have unapologetically embraced their age, their wrinkles and their weight were displaying their years with such magnificence that I would have traded my youthful, pain-free body and life, there and then, just to be part of their irresistible trinity.

They were dressed with that flamboyant elegance only Italians know how to create.

They smoked cigarettes.

They laughed.

They shared a bottle of white wine and appetisers.

They flirted with the waiter, and the waiter flirted back.

They laughed some more.

They ate heartily.

They asked for some water for the Dachshund accompanying them. The dog sported a chic orange leather collar with a silver clasp.

They ordered another bottle of wine.

They were not loud, but I remember there was something deliciously extravagant about them.

I didn't understand a word they said, but I understood that they were unapologetic about the way they lived their life, and each of them seemed to be living it as if it was her last hour on earth.

For the first time in my life, 'older' looked anything but old, and I remember thinking: 'Life doesn't have to end at fifty or sixty... You can still create, and have fun, and fall in love and be rebellious and dance and have dreams and remain totally cool doing it. When am older I want to be just like these women.'

When I am older is now.

As a matter of fact, it's been *when I am older* for quite some time now, and looking back, I realise this indelible scene, which Federico Fellini could very well have directed, captured to perfection the fundamental traits of a blossoming post-menopausal life.

And so, based on this lasting memory, my personal

experience with menopause and comprehensive research, I decided to compile a list of ingredients that seem to be common denominators for women living well after menopause.

Firstly, I discovered that the perfect, sacred guide to post-menopausal happiness (and to life in general) doesn't exist, so I quickly established that women do not menopause and live happily ever after.

I did find out something else, though. Something better.

So here is an unassuming testimony of the silver linings of post-menopausal life, and probably the source of the poignant vitality I witnessed circa 1995 with this unforgettable Fellini sequence.

The following chapters provide solace.

No really… they do.

NO MORE PERIODS. PERIOD.

Ladies (and gentlemen), Carrie has left the building!

After about 400–500 rounds of relentless periods, you are finally done with this monthly exasperation. Your hormonal life may have gone through a serious transformation, but it has also dropped this *bloody* hassle in the process.

I mean, imagine if despite menopausing we were still getting our period!

PMS now stands for POST-MENSTRUAL SALVATION. Savour it!

No more pads or tampons on your shopping list, no more bleeding guessing game before your summer holidays, no more 'Oh sh*t, I think I'm getting my period' in the middle of a crowded mall with the nearest toilet a mile away.

No more protected sex, too – assuming your libido has survived the menopausal laws of fornication, and that your partner is not some shady character you stumbled upon just before the pub's closing time.

In that case you still need protection.

Maybe a little emotional reflection wouldn't hurt either here.

For the rest of us, let's recognise the blessings when they cross our paths, for we will never ever miss the practical details of menstruation.

A SENSE OF HUMOUR FOR A SENSE OF SELF

If I don't laugh, I die.

If I don't laugh at myself, I die even more.

My father was a man who liked to laugh a lot and who happened to be extremely funny and sharp. The darker the situation, the more dazzling the witticisms, and the larger the laughs.

For as long as I can remember, this approach has helped my siblings and me to defuse so many painful situations. Humour has somewhat protected us from life's glitches, and even from ourselves at times.

We've always tried not to take life too seriously, even when it was dead serious.

Looking back, I realise I have always surrounded myself with genuinely funny people who understand the vital significance of having a good sense of humour and *a life well laughed...* with one exception.

Those particularly close to me also know that my speciality has always been poking fun at myself – and God knows that over the years, life has provided me with some honest material for this.

But wait.

My self-deprecation is not self-derogatory; I just like to laugh. It's not about low self-esteem or insecurity, either, and it's certainly not about making fun of myself before someone else does; I just really like to laugh.

There's another explanation, though – other than me being a giggling hyena.

I am, alas, a bit of a drama queen too. I speak tragicomedy fluently. I am gifted with such a vivid imagination when creating worst-case scenarios that I sometimes wonder if I am actually all OK in there, and my emotional energy when I am in distress can be quite incapacitating at times.

I also cry easily and I am exceptionally sensitive. I get very excited about tiny little things, and anxious about tiny little things too. It's fair to say that my sponge heart is often in command.

Fortunately, with age, the intensity of my colourful personality has softened considerably, but imagine a life lived with all the above-mentioned traits and no sense of humour?

On a scale of one to Shakespeare, life would be an insufferable nine point five.

I would basically *not be*.

We can't always control our sorrows and insecurities, but when we laugh at life or ourselves, it often helps us attain some distance from the upsetting situation (and from ourselves in the process). From a comical angle, it's so much easier to assess and rationalise the complications of life more objectively.

Some call it a peculiar coping mechanism, others a snap-out-of-it remedy; all I know is that it's one of the most efficient and healthy responses to the glitches and hitches of our existence I have found.

A well-functioning sense of humour has the power to de-dramatise the most dramatic situation. It's a great way to fight stress and anxiety; it brings people closer together; and it gives you a different perspective on everything in life.

Also, let's not forget endorphins, please.

So, when it came to menopause – before, during and after – I took the same route, and instead of letting its ravaging symptoms have the last laugh, I did.

Have the last laugh.

Hahaha…

MENOPAUSE PRIORITIES 2.0

1. I'm sorry, I won't be able to attend your cousin's abstract exhibition tonight; I must watch *Dahmer* and cuddle with my cat.
2. This is me, take it or leave it.
3. Yes, I just sent you a message on WhatsApp. No, I will not answer your phone call. Yes, I am still holding my phone and appear to be online. No, I still won't answer.
4. Pizza gives me heartburn. Yes, I am going to eat this pizza.
5. I don't want to FaceTime and hear the details of your urinary tract infection again – I'm busy taking an online test to see if I'm an empath.
6. No, I am not willing to stay an extra hour at work to help you with your filing. I have to go home and sit on the sofa.
7. Roses are red, violets are blue. Am so done putting me after you.
8. Apologies for not showing up yesterday. Nope, no reason at all.

9. I'm sorry I didn't show more enthusiasm about your Botox and filler injections – as it turns out, I don't really care.
10. If you need me, remember, I'm always seven missed calls away.

#JESUISKAREN

'Don't be a Karen, Mum...'

By Mum, he means me.

I wasn't going to come out with a vile tirade of 'I want to speak to the manager... do you know who I am... this rule doesn't apply to me', etcetera.

I was just going to politely and legitimately ask the waiter, who had seated us over fifteen minutes ago, if we could please have the menu, and voluntarily omit to mention the fact that he had taken the orders of two tables of people that arrived after us, thank you very much.

If that makes me a Karen, then hand me a whistle and drop me in the middle of the busiest street in town – I'm open for business!

There was a time when I would have sat silently and docilely waiting for the waiter to acknowledge my presence, no matter how long it took him. Not because I am shy or weak; I used to let it go in the name of being the bigger person, on account of my empathy.

For decades I kept my mouth shut because I didn't

want to escalate things or hurt the other person's feelings or draw attention to myself. I still don't want things to escalate, and I definitely don't want to hurt anybody's feelings, but when menopause arrived something happened.

It suddenly felt as if my biological stock of patience, sacrifice and compromise had been sucked dry, and one morning I simply decided I had performed my fair share of magnanimity in this lifetime and on this planet.

I didn't want to be the bigger person anymore, and I couldn't help it if I tried.

I can't stand it when the waiter serves you attitude along with your coffee, or when people jump the queue and pretend they didn't see you and the other seven people standing in line. I get frustrated when a young man doesn't offer his seat to a pregnant woman or an old man on the bus, despite noticing their presence; or when the salesperson in a high-end designer store is arrogant and rude to a customer because her look doesn't conform to the *ladies who lunch* style.

I can't stand staying silent in the face of prejudice anymore, no matter how tiny the action may be, because I realised that every time I kept quiet to avoid a fight on the outside, I triggered a fight in my insides.

So now I speak my mind and point out the obvious when people are unkind, unfair, offensive or disrespectful.

And then it hit me. I had become a Karen.

A courteous and humane but firm, fair and blunt Karen.

The waiter brought the menu with an apology and a smile. Flawless service ensued.

I tipped him generously and thanked him profusely too.
My son still thinks I'm a Karen.

I PLEAD NOT GUILTY

For decades, and on an almost daily basis, guilt has crept into every aspect of our lives, sometimes becoming as instinctive as thirst or hunger. *Was I too honest? Was I too compliant? Did I do the right thing? Is this dress too revealing? Am I thin enough? Good enough?* At times, we even felt guilty about feeling guilty!

But after a lifetime of self-critical female kryptonite feasting on our confidence and tricking our minds into thinking we could have been better daughters, dancers, bakers, mothers, drivers, yogis, wives, employees, friends, neighbours, hostesses, etcetera, we have now come to the conclusion that we did our best, and quite frankly our best was good enough.

Our best was even borderline *bestest* at times.

An uplifting incentive most women I know have experienced and welcomed with the onset of menopause is the unexpected realisation that guilt has lost its supremacy over their conscience and their lives.

We were told that skipping a few football matches (out

of fifty games a year) to have a mimosa-fuelled brunch with our girlfriends was called selfishness, when in fact it was called self-preservation.

We believed that when we weren't working, cleaning, hosting or on mum duty, we had to look like one of Madame Claude's girls, and if we didn't (and often we didn't…) we felt unfeminine, insecure, unlovable, threatened. Even if all along we were responsible for the fundamental structure of our household and for every family member's wellbeing.

We were made to think that we were missing out on our children's best years if we were working mothers, and that we were dull and uninteresting if we were stay-at-home mums or housewives. The reality was that we weren't missing out and we weren't boring. We just had to make choices and stick to them, and we did.

With experience, maturity, age, life, and, well… menopause, we know today that this guilt was toxic, with a pH level of 0.00001!

I for one have dropped this fraudulent feeling for good.

I don't feel guilty about being lazy at times or saying no. I don't feel any kind of remorse about skipping an event I've been invited to simply because the thought of sitting at home, bra-less, in my ugly tracksuit covered in crisp crumbs is more appealing than a dress, makeup and small talk. I don't feel guilty for not showing any interest in a conversation that doesn't interest me, or about not being the perfect daughter, dancer (to be determined), baker, mother, driver, friend, neighbour or hostess; because I have genuinely come to the conclusion that I did my best and that quite frankly my best was good enough.

My best was even borderline *bestest* at times.

PS: Dictionaries define *guilty* as having committed an offense, a crime, a violation, or something wrong, especially against moral or penal law.

VALID REASONS TO FEEL GUILTY

1. You spent your straight-A child's college fund on the Empathy Suite at the Palms Casino Resort in Las Vegas at $100,000 a night because you were feeling spontaneous. And also, you're an empath… and the suite's name is Empathy… and if that's not a sign from destiny right there, then you don't know what is.
2. You keep on flirting with Eddy the hot thirty-something pool guy with an incredible Māori tattoo on his tanned chest while, deliberately knowing that your libido will not put its money where your mouth is.
3. You vaped in a plane toilet, because somehow you are still convinced it's OK to vape indoors, and believe vaping doesn't even smell – every single non-vaping friend who assures you it really stinks is a liar.

4. You smashed up your husband's brand-new phone because it's Valentine's day and he only got you one rose. The fact that you specifically insisted he didn't get you anything this year is totally irrelevant.
5. You drank yourself stupid and offered to drop off your friends on your way home, despite the fact that you are completely plastered. Also, you are the one hosting them.
6. You swiped the little blue porcelain dolphin from your therapist's desk while he was busy getting your file. The file about your persistent sense of guilt… and your kleptomania.
7. You ransacked the McDonald's counter after poor Jenny, who's on her first day working there, said she couldn't serve you an Egg McMuffin and McPancakes. It's 2pm.
8. You were involved in theft, drug crime, aggravated assault or murder.
9. You peed in a swimming pool. Unforgivable – you should be ashamed of yourself. Criminal, really. Have you no soul?

BUDDY BODY

Who hasn't gone through this time distortion?

You look at a picture of yourself dated two years ago and can't believe how skinny you were, only to remember that at the time you thought you were fat.

I wasted a big part of my life running after a weight that kept on slipping between my brain cells every time I reached it.

I was never thin enough, even when the scale screamed the opposite. My body was never fit enough, even if I worked out two hours a day, seven days a week, and I was convinced that not being a skeleton was the source of all my life's problems.

When I lose weight, I will do *everything and then some*, was my mantra.

Eventually, I would go that dangerous extra mile called an eating disorder, and spend years battling bulimia.

It would take me another few years to free myself from this mental disorder and reconcile with food, body and self.

Ironically, I started loving my body when it became subjected to cruel scrutiny and denigration, which coincided with the exact time menopause landed in my life. That was when it became clear it was my sole responsibility to respect my body and be kind to it, no matter how it looked or how much it weighed; when I understood that this incredibly sophisticated organism had a purpose other than vanity and the desperate need to have people love ~~it~~ me.

Menopause and age come with certain pitfalls, that is undeniable, but there is a sense of comfort and kindness in growing older – a feeling that this massive and unreasonable pressure many women feel to look perfect has been lifted.

Sure, I may be heavier than I was two years ago, five years ago, or twenty years ago, but my heart and my mind have never felt so light. I certainly won't hate myself for not having a perfect body anymore.

Some call it carelessness. I call it self-love.

THE URGENCY OF A BUCKET LIST

Every woman, once she reaches fifty, should sit in front of a blank piece of paper and ask herself: *what do I really want to do and experience before I die?*

Every woman, once she reaches fifty, should write down a non-negotiable, greedy, unapologetic, crazy-if-it-needs-to-be list of all the long-lost dreams, pent-up foolishness and absurd aspirations she has ignored or neglected during her life so far.

A list harnessing the power of now, because tomorrow her body or mind could decide that she can't do these things anymore.

Every woman in her fifties should have a bucket list.

I once made a bucket list, back when I was younger.

At the time, I was convinced my little inventory was outrageous, wild and exceptional, when in reality it was filled with textbook bucket-list material, probably shared by 80% of people who have bucket lists.

I wanted to swim with dolphins, skydive, see the northern lights, learn hip-hop dancing, scream at the top of one of the highest places in the world (like a small Swiss mountain) and get a tattoo, among other predictable aspirations an ordinary twenty-something woman with a pinch of ennui and a total lack of imagination would entertain.

I shared my list with my brother once, and after listening to his older sister's puerile aspirations, he pointed out that it sounded a lot like your typical tourist bucket list, and that if I really wanted, I could cover 80% of it in Dubai… in one day!

I have done many things since making that list.

I paraglided, I saved a life, I jumped off a cliff, I went rafting, I met a healer (no, for real). I did things that were brave, others that were reckless, and many that were human.

I am not done yet.

I still want to skydive, swim with dolphins, see the northern lights and get a tattoo, but with age, my list has become more heartfelt than ever (I have had three decades to think about it, after all). It also has a sense of urgency chained to it now.

My list has got longer, too, and doesn't only include risky adventures and extraordinary challenges. It contains feelings as well, connections and reconnections, simplicity, kindness, and closure. It contains my life.

It remains as cliché and unoriginal as ever, though.

ANATOMY OF A BUCKET LIST FOR WOMEN OVER FIFTY

Any respectable bucket list should have:

Something to give and forgive
An old designer bag sleeping in your closet? A four-year-old foldable exercise bike still in its box? Give them a second life; give them away to someone who will find pleasure in wearing or using them. Give a total stranger a compliment (in real life). Why be shy? We do it on Instagram every day. Repeat indefinitely if you find pleasure in it.

*For*give, too. Don't hold grudges.

Your mother-in-law's been getting involved in your business again? Forgive her – there's no time for resentment. Your husband forgot your wedding anniversary? Forgive him – there's no harm done.

Your ex-husband/ex-girlfriend/ex-boss was toxic? ~~Forgive~~ Find something else to forgive.

Something crazy
Don't settle for painting, piano, pottery, knitting and book clubs. Do you really want to know what the lady in the green cardigan sitting opposite you thinks of *It is a truth universally acknowledged, that a single man in possession of a good fortune, must be in want of a wife* while munching on mushroom quiche? Honestly.

Try pole dancing, hip hop, acting, spelling bees… Pick a hobby where you are least expected to show up, and show up. Nobody should put you in a corner.

Get a tattoo. (Yes, I am projecting here.)

Something audacious
Go skinny dipping. Fine, you can keep the bottom half on…

Go to a full-house Karaoke night and sing your favourite song with your whole body, heart and soul. Sing it like nobody is listening. Be silly. Seriously, when was the last time you were silly?

Something scary
Go skydiving. No, you're not too old. Swedish woman Rut Linnéa Ingegärd Larsson did it at 103. (Not metres. Years old.)

Swim with sharks if the idea of swimming with dolphins isn't scary enough.

Swim in iced water if the idea of swimming with sharks isn't scary enough.

And if the idea of swimming in iced water isn't scary enough, swim with dolphins and sharks in iced water.

At night.

Something meaningful

Tell your mama and your papa you love them. As many times as you can. The older they get, the more they need to hear it, despite the grumpy façade. Tell your siblings, too, and your friends. Tell them often.

Tell your kids you really did your best.

Tell yourself you did your best, too.

Something challenging

Run a mini/half/full marathon.

Read Marcel Proust's *In Search of Lost Time*… all 3,408 pages and six volumes. (Not to brag or anything, but I did.)

Solve a 2000-piece jigsaw puzzle – do something that requires dedication, consistency, patience, and fortitude.

Surpass yourself; surprise yourself. You still can.

Something high

Climb a tree, a mountain, a tower, Kilimanjaro. Pick something that will take you high enough – there's something terribly exhilarating about that altitude and angle.

No, marijuana doesn't count.

Something fun

Go on an Italian holiday with your besties (rent the Vespas, eat the pasta, dance the tarantella…). Go on a themed picnic, if that's more accessible. Go dancing with your friends. Be the oldest ones in the club. You and the creepy Peter-Pan fifty-year-old regulars out there.

Celebrate life and friendship. Together.

Something beautiful

Stop saving beauty for a special occasion. Use your fine china and crystal glasses daily; wear your new clothes to the supermarket; open that Châteauneuf-du-Pape; light the exclusive Dyptique candle. Don't feel guilty or undeserving. Don't wait for the special occasion – create the special occasion.

Something simple

Sit under a tree, breathe in the aroma of the sunrise, take a long, restful bath, indulge in that piece of chocolate cake, listen to blaring music, dance with yourself... and do it mindfully.

Things done mindfully taste, feel, smell, look and sound different – better.

OLDER WOMEN ARE HAPPIER WOMEN

Older women are happier women.

They have exorcised their inner demons. They know themselves now, and have encountered this beautiful thing called wisdom along the way. They express anger, joy, fear and sadness, because they understand that keeping it in is poisonous. They have developed an aversion to poison.

Older women don't need to be loved by everyone anymore. They know it's impossible to be loved by everyone. Their relationships are open and genuinely based on the age-old maxim *it's the beauty within that matters*. The beauty within was all that mattered all along – they know that now.

They have grown more compassionate, and ironically have learned to be more selfish too.

They know when to use *which* and *with whom*.

Older women are happier women.

They take their time. They see the splendour in a tree and tear up; they sense the wind blowing on a deserted beach and smile; they inhale the warmth of coffee in the morning and are grateful; they can sit and listen to a sonata, and do only that, because they appreciate that listening to a sonata is an endeavour all of its own. They dissociate for a second or two while at dinner with family or friends, just to say 'thank you, life,' and then dive back into the blessed moment.

Older women are happier women.

They sometimes feel like their life is one big extraordinary failure, and that they should have done more and been more.

But they know this feeling has nothing to do with their actual life; that it's just a momentary groundless doubt.

They have done their best.

They are their best.

Older women are happier women.

They have forgiven and accepted. They see a full glass, greener grass, a sky full of stars. They no longer add anything harmful after the word *self*.

Self comes with love, esteem, expression, consideration. The self is protected. At last.

Older women are happier women.

They look at newborns with tenderness, and compassion, too. They know the road will be long and there will be plenty of turbulence along the way for these minuscule beings.

They know that in the end it will be OK.

They are glad they are not newborns.

Older women are happier women.

They know that happiness is nothing but a fleeting moment.

And so is life.

TO BELONG AT LAST

I became an eating disorder recovery coach because when bulimia was my unshakeable belief system, finding comfort, answers or a safe space was a distinctly challenging affair.

At the time, deliberately throwing up the thousand calories you had just swallowed wasn't something you shared with people, no matter how close to them you were.

Bulimia is severely misunderstood, because it involves food and many women have a somewhat complicated relationship with food. Most women I know enjoy food; they have all wished at some point in their lives that their thighs were a bit slimmer; and all of them have refrained at least once from indulging in that inviting piece of cake when summer was imminent.

This is probably the reason why so many people assume that bulimics are just ordinary people who can't control their food intake. Which, theoretically, is true, but the reason they can't is not because they are weak or don't have the willpower, determination or desire. Bulimics have all of these and then some.

Bulimics cannot control their food intake because bulimia is an addiction. And like any addiction, it controls you.

Recovery is hard, but I recovered, and once I did, it became the most logical, natural next step to help other women do the same.

Giving them what I wasn't given, holding the hand that their illness had pulled towards isolation, and showing their hearts the way out became one of the most meaningful journeys of my life, after raising my two beautiful boys.

My main aspiration was to help them realise that they were not alone, that they weren't mad, and that somewhere, some time ago, someone else had walked the same desperate path they were trapped on now.

Which, in retrospect, I realised closely resembled the complicated journey that is menopause.

Menopause has many layers. It can isolate, hurt and frighten, and while unlike an eating disorder it is a natural occurrence, it does at times seem to hijack your life and identity just like an eating disorder.

I genuinely believe that from birth to death, women share one intricate and fascinating emotional, physical, and hormonal journey – menopause being the coronation of all its stages.

Mothers, daughters, wives, beekeepers, social butterflies, artists, acrobats, housewives; rich, poor, thin, petite, overweight, blonde, brunette; no matter the race, country, religion or walk of life, I am persuaded that together we are not necessarily stronger, but we are less alone.

We belong.

THE BEGINNING OF THE END IS STILL A BEGINNING

I menopaused ten years ago exactly.

To say it has been one chaotic journey would be the understatement of the decade.

During these ten years, I have hot flashed thousands of times; gained weight and lost it, and gained it again and lost it again; suffered from insomnia and digestive issues; developed arthritis, or osteoporosis (I'm still not sure which is which); lost my hair, my home, my mind, my sex appeal, my dignity at times, my libido, my temper (although some people really deserved it) and my groove (still to be determined); got dumped; suffered from depression; hit rock bottom and discovered it had a basement; experienced empty-nest syndrome, twice; questioned my life, my choices, myself; lost hope many times; let myself down even more times; and, to reiterate, hot flashed thousands of times.

But I also understood the power of self-acceptance, of forgiveness, and of gratitude, too. I overcame bulimia; quit smoking; got therapy; became an eating disorder recovery coach and still love every single second of it; met fascinating women along the way; realised that I was never really alone and that there are some incredible souls out there; reconnected with my childhood; and became financially independent.

I discovered my infinite love for nature and God, understood the power of family and truth, and managed to *once upon a time* myself after fifty…

…Oh, and I wrote a little book I called *Menopostal*.

PS: For those of you suddenly wondering why their menopause is not a happy-go-lucky adventure, please Keep Calm and stop the self-flagellation immediately.

While *Menopostal* concludes on a whoopee note, I obviously did not live happily ever after.

Nobody does.

Wait… maybe Patsy and Eddie did.

Yeah, these *Absolutely Fabulous* women absolutely did.

ACKNOWLEDGEMENTS

To my pillars of love during the writing of this little book, thank you, thank you, thank you…

First and foremost, to my sister, Ghada, who one afternoon, upon receiving from me – for no particular reason – a small piece I had written about menopause hot flashes, strongly suggested that I turn this random rambling into a book.

To my dear friend Jayne Mayer, who, along with my sister, has read each chapter as it was written and offered her precious encouragement every time I would say, "I'm not sure… do you really think it's any good?"

A special word of thanks to my editor, Laura Shanahan, who meticulously reviewed my manuscript. I am also indebted to my dear friend and talented author, Nadia Wassef, for her generous feedback and kind support throughout the writing process.

To Mamouche, my mother, a role model of menopausal resilience. And resilience.

To my siblings, Fafo and Khaled, for their tireless encouragement in everything I do or try to do.

To the incredible Menopostal women of my life: Nathalie Lasnon, Mona Elyafi, Sherry Youssef, Lara Zureikat, Julia Assaad, Nabila Massrali, Marine Auger, Heba Shunbo, and Cécile Bedoian. You have always been an infinite source of admiration and motivation – before, during, and after menopause.

To my nieces Lara and Sara, I hope this book will remain relevant decades from now and serve as an instrument of laughter and fortitude when you face the challenges of menopause.

To my precious boys, Hussein and Youssef – you are the driving force behind this little book and my life.

Last but not least, to my late Baba, thank you for instilling in me your love for words and laughter and fostering my passion for storytelling.

This book is printed on paper from sustainable sources managed under the Forest Stewardship Council (FSC) scheme.

It has been printed in the UK to reduce transportation miles and their impact upon the environment.

For every new title that Troubador publishes, we plant a tree to offset CO_2, partnering with the More Trees scheme.

MORE TREES
LET'S PLANT A BILLION TREES

For more about how Troubador offsets its environmental impact, see www.troubador.co.uk/sustainability-and-community